MEDICATION SAFETY IN PREGNANCY AND BREASTFEEDING

The Evidence-Based,
A-to-Z Clinician's Pocket Guide

NOTICE

Medicine is an ever-changing science. As new research and clinical experience broaden our knowledge, changes in treatment and drug therapy are required. The authors and the publisher of this work have checked with sources believed to be reliable in their efforts to provide information that is complete and generally in accord with the standards accepted at the time of publication. However, in view of the possibility of human error or changes in medical sciences, neither the authors nor the publisher nor any other party who has been involved in the preparation or publication of this work warrants that the information contained herein is in every respect accurate or complete, and they disclaim all responsibility for any errors or omissions or for the results obtained from use of the information contained in this work. Readers are encouraged to confirm the information contained herein with other sources. For example, and in particular, readers are advised to check the product information sheet included in the package of each drug they plan to administer to be certain that the information contained in this work is accurate and that changes have not been made in the recommended dose or in the contraindications for administration. This recommendation is of particular importance in connection with new or infrequently used drugs.

MEDICATION SAFETY IN PREGNANCY AND BREASTFEEDING

The Evidence-Based, A-to-Z Clinician's Pocket Guide

Gideon Koren, MD, FRCPC

Director and Professor, Motherisk Program,
    The Hospital for Sick Children;
Professor of Pediatrics, Pharmacology, Pharmacy,
    & Medical Genetics, University of Toronto;
Richard and Jean Ivey Chair in Molecular Toxicology,
    Schulich School of Medicine,
The University of Western Ontario

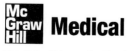

Medical

New York   Chicago   San Francisco   Lisbon   London   Madrid   Mexico City
Milan   New Delhi   San Juan   Seoul   Singapore   Sydney   Toronto

The McGraw·Hill Companies

MEDICATION SAFETY IN PREGNANCY & BREASTFEEDING:
The Evidence-Based, A-to-Z Clinician's Pocket Guide

1 2 3 4 5 6 7 8 9 0   DOC/DOC   0 9 8 7 6

ISBN 13: 978-0-07-110059-5
ISBN 10: 0-07-144827-6

This book was set in Souvenir by International Typesetting and Composition.
The editors were James F. Shanahan and Maya Barahona.
The production supervisor was Sherri Souffrance.
Project Management was provided by International Typesetting and Composition.
The index was prepared by Robert Swanson.
RR Donnelley was the printer and binder.
This book is printed on acid-free paper.

Library of Congress Cataloging-in-Publication Data

Medication safety in pregnancy & breastfeeding: A to Z pocket guide / [edited by] Gideon Koren.—1st ed.
   P. ; cm.
   Includes bibliographical references and index.
   ISBN 0-07-144827-6 (softcover:alk.paper)
   1. Fetus—Effect of drugs on—Handbooks, manuals, etc.   2. Infants (Newborn)—Effect of drugs on—Handbooks, manuals, etc.   3. Breast milk—Contamination—Handbooks, manuals, etc.   4. Drugs—Side effects—Handbooks, manuals, etc.   I. Koren, Gideon, 1947–.   II. Title: Medication safety in pregnancy and breastfeeding.
   [DNLM: 1. Drug Toxicity—Handbooks.   2. Pregnancy—drug effects—Handbooks.   3. Breast Feeding—Handbooks.   4. Pharmaceutical Preparations—adverse effects—Handbooks.   WQ 39 M488   2007]
RG627.6.D79M4344   2007
618.3'2686—dc22   2006028764

INTERNATIONAL EDITION ISBN-13: 978-0-07-110059-5; ISBN-10: 0-07-110059-8

This book is dedicated to
my parents,
wife,
children,
and grandchildren.

CONTENTS

CONTRIBUTORS

Facundo Garcia-Bournissen, MD
Clinical Fellow
Division of Clinical Pharmacology
and Toxicology
The Hospital for Sick Children
University of Toronto
Ontario, Canada

Adrienne Einarson, RN
Assistant Director
The Motherisk Program
The Hospital for Sick Children
University of Toronto
Ontario, Canada

Cameron J. Gilbert, MSc
Graduate Student
Institute of Medical Science
University of Toronto
The Motherisk Program
Division of Clinical Pharmacology
and Toxicology
The Hospital for Sick Children
Ontario, Canada

Ran D. Goldman, MD
Associate Professor
Department of Pediatrics
Division of Pediatric
Emergency Medicine and
Clinical Pharmacology
and Toxicology
The Hospital for Sick Children
University of Toronto
Ontario, Canada

Shinya Ito, MD
Professor and Head
Division of Clinical Pharmacology
and Toxicology
Department of Pediatrics
The Hospital for Sick Children
University of Toronto
Ontario, Canada

Sanjog Kalra, MSc
Graduate Student
Department of Pharmacology
University of Toronto
The Motherisk Program
Division of Clinical Pharmacology
and Toxicology
The Hospital for Sick Children
University of Toronto
Ontario, Canada

Debra Kennedy, MBBS, FRACP
Director and Clinical Geneticist,
MotherSafe
Royal Hospital for Women
Randwick, Australia
Conjoint Lecturer
Women's and Children's Health
University of New South Wales
Sydney, Australia

Eran Kozer, MD
Pediatric Emergency Service
Assaf Harefeh Medical Center
Sackler School of Medicine
Tel Aviv University
Tel Aviv, Israel

Michael Lishner, MD

Professor
Meir Medical Center
Kfar Saba and Sackler Faculty
of Medicine
Tel Aviv University
Tel Aviv, Israel

Caroline Maltepe, BA

NVP Helpline Coordinator
The Motherisk Program
Department of Clinical
Pharmacology and Toxicology
The Hospital for Sick Children
University of Toronto
Ontario, Canada

Ariel Many, MD, MHA

Lis Maternity Hospital
Tel Aviv Sourasky Medical Center
Tel Aviv University
Israel

Myla Moretti, MSc

Assistant Director
The Motherisk Program
Project Director
The Research Institute
The Hospital for Sick Children
University of Toronto
Ontario, Canada

Irena Nulman, MD

Associate Professor
Department of Pediatrics
University of Toronto
Associate Director
The Motherisk Program
The Hospital for Sick Children
University of Toronto
Ontario, Canada

Alejandro A. Nava-Ocampo, MD

The Motherisk Program
Division of Clinical Pharmacology
and Toxicology
The Hospital for Sick Children
and PharmaReasons, Toronto
Ontario, Canada

Lavinia Schüler-Faccini, MD, PhD

Associate Professor
Department of Genetics
School of Medicine
Federal University of Rio Grande
do Sul
Porto Alegre, Brazil

Alon Shrim, MD

The Motherisk Program
Division of Clinical Pharmacology
and Toxicology
The Hospital for Sick Children
University of Toronto
Ontario, Canada

Samar R. Shuhaiber, MSc

Drug Information Associate
Apotex, Inc., Toronto
Ontario, Canada

PREFACE

Establishing the safety of medications in pregnancy is one of the most challenging tasks for the practicing physician. With about fifty percent of all pregnancies unplanned, large numbers of women are seeing their health care providers in high levels of anxiety after unintentionally taking medications or recreational drugs into pregnancy. Yet another large group of pregnant women must continue to take medications for chronic conditions such as epilepsy or diabetes, or for pregnancy-induced conditions such as hypertension or morning sickness.

For many medications, the available evidence is sparse. Yet, very often, even where there is large knowledge base, drug companies are reluctant to support the use of their products in pregnancy due to fear of litigation; hence, the text in the Physician Desk Reference or the Compendium of Pharmaceuticals and Specialties is not supportive.

For decades, much of the world has used the FDA system of teratogenic risk, ranging from A (definitely safe) to X (definitely contra indicated). However, this system has been widely criticized as ambiguous and clinically unhelpful. For example, the oral contraceptive pill, which is by far the most common prescribed agent women are exposed to in pregnancy (due to contraception failure), has been labeled until recently as an X, despite repeated studies and two meta analyses failing to show teratogenic risk in the doses currently used. Critically, when evaluating teratogenic risk it is critical to consider the risks to the mother and fetus of the untreated maternal condition.

In this A-to-Z Pocket Guide, we offer a novel and different approach to counseling on drugs and chemicals. It is based on the method developed by the Motherisk Program at the Hospital for Sick Children and the University of Toronto (*www.motherisk.org*). Since 1985 Motherisk has counseled and informed hundreds of thousands of pregnant women, their families and health care professionals. The information is based on ongoing evaluation of all existing data, for both pregnancy and lactation.

This book acknowledges that busy clinicians are not likely to be able to read large texts during patient encounters, and hence the A-to-Z

Pocket Guide concentrates on the clinical "bottom line." Not only does the Guide include a listing of major drugs with summaries of the known risks, it contains a unique collection of specific clinical questions asked of us over the years by both patients and health care professionals seeking consultations. These specific clinical questions are answered within the Guide with concise answers based upon clinical evidence. (For more comprehensive reviews of critical issues in maternal-fetal prescribing and toxicology, please see Koren G. Medication Safety in Pregnancy and Breastfeeding. New York: McGraw-Hill. In Press.)

I wish to acknowledge and extend thanks to my colleagues at the Motherisk team in Toronto for their daily dedication to the health of pregnant women and their unborn babies; to the Hospital for Sick Children for their unconditional support of this unique program; to the Research Leadership for Better Drugs during Pregnancy and Lactation; and to the Ivey Chair in Molecular Toxicology at the University of Western Ontario. The original research presented herein was supported by the following agencies: Canadian Institutes for Health Research Physician Services Inc, Health Canada, National Institute of Health, March of Dimes, Organization of Teratology Information Services, Mead Johnson Canada, Wal-Mart Canada, the Brewers Association of Canada, Duchesnay Inc., and Novartis Global Epidemiology.

Gideon Koren MD, FRCPC

PART I

RULES OF THUMB FOR TAKING DRUGS DURING PREGNANCY AND BREASTFEEDING

CHAPTER 1

TAKING DRUGS DURING PREGNANCY: HOW SAFE ARE THE UNSAFE?

Gideon Koren, MD, FRCPC
Lavinia Schüler-Faccini, MD, PhD

QUESTION

I prescribed misoprostol to one of my patients with a peptic ulcer. When she found out she was pregnant while on the drug, both she and, admittedly, I were very scared to learn that the drug is teratogenic in that it causes Möbius syndrome. How great is the risk?

Answer

Very small, although women who use misoprostol during the first trimester have a 30-fold higher risk of having babies with Möbius syndrome. The malformation is so rare that, even if you see 1000 women who took misoprostol during embryogenesis, you might not see a single child with the syndrome. It is crucial to explain the size of the risk; otherwise women tend to believe the risk is huge even when, in fact, it is hardly measurable.

Ever since it was discovered in the late 1950s that thalidomide caused fetal malformations, women and health professionals have commonly believed that every drug is potentially harmful to a fetus. When asked, even women exposed to nonteratogenic drugs believe they have a 25% risk of having children with major malformations, apparently the size of the risk with thalidomide itself.[1] This unrealistic perception leads pregnant women to avoid medications even when they clearly need them.[2]

Teratogenicity in humans is studied in different ways. It is important for physicians to understand the advantages and limitations of certain types of studies, so they can inform patients not just whether there is increased risk, but also of the magnitude of that risk.

Cohort studies focus on finding the proportion of children who are malformed after exposure to a certain drug and comparing it with the proportion in an unexposed group. For example, Motherisk recently showed that rates of major malformations among babies born to women exposed occupationally to organic solvents were significantly higher than in a control group consisting of women not working with these chemicals.[3]

Because major malformations occur in 1% to 3% of the general population and any particular malformation is rare, it is not easy to prove that a specific malformation is caused by a specific drug. A much more sensitive method is a case-control study because it focuses on a specific child with a specific malformation.

In a study conducted in Brazil, we showed that children born with Möbius syndrome (facial paralysis and anomalies such as limb deformities) were 30 times more likely to have been exposed to misoprostol in utero than children with other malformations, such as neural tube defects.[4] In Brazil, where therapeutic abortion is illegal, young women use misoprostol as an abortifacient. An odds ratio of 30 sounds scary, but Möbius syndrome is so rare in the general population (one in 50,000 to 100,000 births) that even an odds ratio of 30 is hardly measurable.

Indeed, a prospective cohort study in Brazil showed that none of 86 women who took misoprostol during the first trimester had children with Möbius syndrome.[5] We think misoprostol most likely causes Möbius deformities through vascular disruption, but the risk is marginal.

REFERENCES

1. Koren G, Bologa M, Long D, Feldman Y, Shear NH. Perception of teratogenic risk by pregnant women exposed to drugs and chemicals during the first trimester. *Am J Obstet Gynecol* 1989;160:1190–4.
2. Koren G, Pastuszak A, Ito S. Drugs in pregnancy. *N Engl J Med* 1998; 338:1128–37.
3. Khattak S, Moghtader G, McMartin K, Barrera M, Kennedy D, Koren G. Pregnancy outcome following gestational exposure to organic solvents: a prospective controlled study. *JAMA* 1999;281:1106–9.
4. Pastuszak AP, Schuller L, Speck-Martins CF, Coelho KE, Cordello SM, Vargas F, et al. Use of misoprostol during pregnancy and Moebius syndrome in infants. *N Engl J Med* 1998;338:1881–5.
5. Schuler L, Pastuszak A, Sanseverino TV, Orioli IM, Brunoni D, Ashton-Prolla P, et al. Pregnancy outcome after exposure to misoprostol in Brazil: a prospective controlled study. *Reprod Toxicol* 1999;13:147–51.

WHICH DRUGS ARE CONTRAINDICATED DURING BREASTFEEDING?: PRACTICE GUIDELINES

Myla Moretti, MSc
Shinya Ito, MD
Gideon Koren, MD, FRCPC

I am breastfeeding now and often need a medication. I am concerned about taking medications that might affect my baby. Are there any guidelines on which drugs are safe?

Answer

Only a few drugs pose a clinically significant risk to breastfed babies. In general, antineoplastics, drugs of abuse, some anticonvulsants, ergot alkaloids, and radiopharmaceuticals should not be taken, and levels of amiodarone, cyclosporine, and lithium should be monitored. There is no question that breastfeeding is best for providing all necessary nutrients to infants for the first 6 months of life. Use of medication while lactating, however, complicates the decision to breastfeed. Fortunately, most drugs are compatible with breastfeeding and do not pose a risk to infants. While certain drugs are traditionally contraindicated for nursing mothers, many of these restrictions are based on theoretical concerns only rather than on evidence or clinical observation. In this update we discuss these contraindicated drugs in light of the practice guidelines of the Motherisk Program.

DRUGS GENERALLY CONSIDERED INCOMPATIBLE WITH BREASTFEEDING

Antineoplastics Anticancer drugs used in chemotherapy are generally considered incompatible with breastfeeding because even very low levels of exposure can prove toxic. If breastfeeding is continued, drug levels in milk and infant plasma, and infant hematologic parameters, must be monitored. Much research is still required in this area, and only limited information is available on some of these agents.

Nine cases of infants breastfed by mothers taking azathioprine (25 to 100 mg/day) appear in the current literature. All infants thrived and had no reported adverse effects.[1-3] Breastfeeding might be possible provided infants are closely monitored. Two cases of cisplatin excretion into milk indicated that patients excrete this drug in varying amounts into milk.[4,5] The outcome of infants exposed to cisplatin through milk are not known. Adverse events, including neutropenia[6] and leukopenia,[7] are reported in two infants whose mothers used cyclophosphamide while breastfeeding.

In a single report, low levels of doxorubicin were found in breast milk[5] although infant outcome was not known. Methotrexate is excreted into milk in minimal amounts,[8] and single weekly doses, such as those used for rheumatoid arthritis maintenance therapy, are unlikely to pose substantial risk to babies. Use of methotrexate for cancer chemotherapy is not recommended for lactating mothers because we do not know how it affects suckling infants.

Anticonvulsants Only a few anticonvulsants are excreted in high concentrations in breast milk. Phenobarbital, ethosuximide, and primidone might result in substantial infant exposure.[9] Close monitoring of infants exposed to phenobarbital is warranted because their blood levels might approach therapeutic levels. Sedation has been observed, and there is potential for withdrawal upon weaning.

Drugs of abuse Generally speaking, all drugs of abuse should be avoided by nursing women. In addition to unnecessary infant exposure, mother's ability to care for their babies while under the influence of such substances becomes an issue.

Heavy alcohol consumption was associated with pseudo Cushing's syndrome in a 4-month-old baby.[10] Ethanol was also associated with decreased milk intake by infants,[11] altered sleep patterns,[12] and slower neurologic development.[13] If mothers drink alcohol, breastfeeding could be withheld temporarily (about 2 to 3 hours per drink) to ensure alcohol levels in the milk have diminished.

Amphetamines have been detected in infant urine following maternal therapy.[14] Nothing is known about maternal amphetamine abuse and its potential effect on nursing infants. Cocaine is excreted into breast milk in notable concentrations; infants might accumulate the drug because they are less able than adults to metabolize it. Cocaine has been detected in infant serum, and toxicity has been reported in some infants.[15,16] Infants exposed to marijuana through breast milk showed a delay in motor development at the age of 1 year.[17] Heroin toxicity has been observed in infants breastfed by mothers abusing heroin, but at therapeutic doses, most opioids, such as morphine, meperidine, methadone, and codeine, are excreted into milk in only minimal amounts[18,19] and are compatible with breastfeeding. Phencyclidine, a potent hallucinogen, has been found in breast milk several weeks after maternal dosing.[20] This is attributable to its long half-life; nursing mothers should be encouraged to avoid it.

Ergot alkaloids   Ergotamine therapy during lactation was associated with ergotism (vomiting, diarrhea, occasional convulsions) in a 1934 publication,[21] but not in a more recent study.[22] We do not know how much of this drug is excreted into milk. Until more data are available, other therapies should be considered for patients requiring headache treatment. Ergonovine is known to reduce serum prolactin levels and might inhibit lactation.[23]

Methylergonovine, used for uterine involution, does not influence milk supply. It is not found in clinically significant amounts in breast milk[24] and can be used safely. Bromocriptine effectively suppresses lactation and, hence, is not compatible with breastfeeding. Also, it could be hazardous to mothers.[25]

Others   Although the drugs listed can be used with caution, safer alternative drugs should be considered first if they exist for the particular indication.

Amiodarone excretion into milk varies from person to person. Nursing infants might ingest up to 50% of the maternal dose (on the basis of weight).[26] Also, infant's thyroid gland amiodarone contains large amounts of iodine that could affect infants' thyroid gland. If the decision is made to continue therapy while breastfeeding, the drug should be monitored in breast milk and infant plasma, as should the infant's thyroid function.

Cyclosporine has been used successfully for several lactating mothers.[3,27,28] Breast-milk levels ranged widely, although infant plasma levels, when detectable, were low. Because cyclosporine is a potent immunosuppressant, however, it should be continued during breast-feeding only if levels in milk and infant serum are monitored.

Similar to amiodarone, lithium concentrations vary greatly in milk. Although amiodarone is contraindicated by many authorities because infant plasma levels can reach one-third to half of maternal levels,[29] the only reported adverse event could not rule out possible effects of in utero exposure.[30] Lithium is an excellent example of a drug that requires monitoring and case-by-case assessment so nursing mothers can be successfully treated.

Cigarette smoking should be minimized while breastfeeding. While second-hand smoke exposure is probably the greater concern, smoking might decrease milk supply and nicotine can be measured in breast milk.[31]

Estrogens found in oral contraceptives have been shown to reduce milk production in some mothers. On the other hand, progestin-only contraceptives are unlikely to affect milk supply. If estrogen-containing contraceptives are to be used, therapy should commence only after maternal milk supply is well established, about 6 weeks after delivery.[32] Infant weight gain can be monitored to ensure sufficient milk is produced.

Radiopharmaceuticals might require temporary cessation of breast-feeding because radioactivity sometimes persists in breast milk for hours or even days. Before procedures, breast milk may be pumped and frozen to be given to infants while breastfeeding is temporarily withheld. In addition, mothers should pump and discard their breast milk while the isotope is still present in order to preserve milk production. Recommendations to patients should be individualized to particular agents. Consultation with a nuclear medicine physician and reading the various literature resources available[33,34] will assist in determining the length of breastfeeding interruption.

REFERENCES

1. Coulam CB, Moyer TP, Jiang NS, et al. Breast-feeding after renal transplantation. *Transplant Proc* 1982;14(3):605–609.
2. Grekas DM, Vasiliou SS, Lazarides AN. Immunosuppressive therapy and breast-feeding after renal transplantation [letter]. *Nephron* 1984;37(1):68.
3. Nyberg G, Haljamae U, Frisenette-Fich C, et al. Breast-feeding during treatment with cyclosporine. *Transplantation* 1998;65(2):253–255.

4. De Vries EG, van der Zee AG, Uges DR, et al. Excretion of platinum into breast milk [letter] [published erratum appears in *Lancet* 1989;1(8641):798]. *Lancet* 1989;1(8636):497.

5. Egan PC, Costanza ME, Dodion P, et al. Doxorubicin and cisplatin excretion into human milk. *Cancer Treat Rep* 1985;69(12):1387–1389.

6. Amato D, Niblett JS. Neutropenia from cyclophosphamide in breast milk [letter]. *Med J Aust* 1977;1(11):383–384.

7. Durodola JI. Administration of cyclophosphamide during late pregnancy and early lactation: a case report. *J Natl Med Assoc* 1979;71(2):165–166.

8. Johns DG, Rutherford LD, Leighton PC, et al. Secretion of methotrexate into human milk. *Am J Obstet Gynecol* 1972;112(7):978–980.

9. Nau H, Kuhnz W, Egger HJ, et al. Anticonvulsants during pregnancy and lactation. Transplacental, maternal and neonatal pharmacokinetics. *Clin Pharmacokinet* 1982;7(6):508–543.

10. Binkiewicz A, Robinson MJ, Senior B. Pseudo-Cushing syndrome caused by alcohol in breast milk. *J Pediatr* 1978;93(6):965–967.

11. Mennella JA, Beauchamp GK. The transfer of alcohol to human milk. Effects on flavor and the infantís behavior. *N Engl J Med* 1991;325(14):981–985.

12. Mennella JA, Gerrish CJ. Effects of exposure to alcohol in motherís milk on infant sleep. *Pediatrics* 1998;101(5):E2.

13. Little RE, Anderson KW, Ervin CH, et al. Maternal alcohol use during breast-feeding and infant mental and motor development at one year. *N Engl J Med* 1989;321(7):425–430.

14. Steiner E, Villen T, Hallberg M, et al. Amphetamine secretion in breast milk. *Eur J Clin Pharmacol* 1984;27(1):123–124.

15. Chasnoff IJ, Lewis DE, Squires L. Cocaine intoxication in a breast-fed infant. *Pediatrics* 1987;80(6):836–838.

16. Chaney NE, Franke J, Wadlington WB. Cocaine convulsions in a breast-feeding baby. *J Pediatr* 1988;112(1):134–135.

17. Astley SJ, Little RE. Maternal marijuana use during lactation and infant development at one year. *Neurotoxicol Teratol* 1990;12(2):161–168.

18. Feilberg VL, Rosenborg D, Broen CC, et al. Excretion of morphine in human breast milk. *Acta Anaesthesiol Scand* 1989;33(5):426–428.

19. Wojnar-Horton RE, Kristensen JH, Yapp P, et al. Methadone distribution and excretion into breast milk of clients in a methadone maintenance programme. *Br J Clin Pharmacol* 1997;44(6):543–547.

20. Kaufman KR, Petrucha RA, Pitts FN Jr, et al. PCP in amniotic fluid and breast milk: case report. *J Clin Psychiatry* 1983;44(7):269–270.

21. Fomina PI. Untersuchungen uber den ubergang des aktiven Agens des Mutterkorns in die milch stillender Mutter. *Arch Gynakol* 1934;157:275–285.

22. Jolivet A, Robyn C, Huraux-Rendu C, et al. Effet de derives des alcaloides de líergot de siegle sur la secretion lactee dans le post-partum immediat [Effect of ergot alkaloid derivatives on milk secretion in the immediate postpartum period] (Fr). *J Gynecol Obstet Biol Reprod (Paris)* 1978;7(1):129–134.

23. Shane JM, Naftolin F. Effect of ergonovine maleate on puerperal prolactin. *Am J Obstet Gynecol* 1974;120(1):129–131.

24. Del Pozo E, Brun DR, Hinselmann M. Lack of effect of methyl-ergonovine on postpartum lactation. *Am J Obstet Gynecol* 1975;123(8):845–846.
25. Comabella M, Alvarez-Sabin J, Rovira A, et al. Bromocriptine and postpartum cerebral angiopathy: a causal relationship? *Neurology* 1996; 46(6):1754–1756.
26. McKenna WJ, Harris L, Rowland E, et al. Amiodarone therapy during pregnancy. *Am J Cardiol* 1983;51(7):1231–1233.
27. Flechner SM, Katz AR, Rogers AJ, et al. The presence of cyclosporine in body tissues and fluids during pregnancy. *Am J Kidney Dis* 1985;5(1): 60–63.
28. Thiru Y, Bateman DN, Coulthard MG. Successful breast feeding while mother was taking cyclosporin. *BMJ* 1997;315(7106):463.
29. Schou M, Amdisen A. Lithium and pregnancy. 3. Lithium ingestion by children breast-fed by women on lithium treatment. *BMJ* 1973;2(859): 138.
30. Tunnessen WW Jr, Hertz CG. Toxic effects of lithium in newborn infants: a commentary. *J Pediatr* 1972;81(4):804–807.
31. Dahlstrom A, Lundell B, Curvall M, et al. Nicotine and cotinine concentrations in the nursing mother and her infant. *Acta Paediatr Scand* 1990;79(2):142–147.
32. Kelsey JJ. Hormonal contraception and lactation [review]. *J Hum Lact* 1996;12(4):315–318.
33. Rubow S, Klopper J, Wasserman H, et al. The excretion of radiopharmaceuticals in human breast milk: additional data and dosimetry. *Eur J Nucl Med* 1994;21(2):144–153.
34. Romney BM, Nickoloff EL, Esser PD, et al. Radionuclide administration to nursing mothers: mathematically derived guidelines. *Radiology* 1986;160(2): 549–554.

CONTINUING DRUG THERAPY WHILE BREASTFEEDING: COMMON MISCONCEPTIONS OF PATIENTS

Shinya Ito, MD
Gideon Koren, MD, FRCPC

QUESTION

Some of my patients who need specific drugs during the postpartum period are hesitant to breastfeed even when I tell them that, according to available evidence, these drugs are safe. Am I right about this and how should I advise my patients?

Answer

Recent studies reveal that women receiving chronic therapy tend to initiate breastfeeding much less often than mothers in the general population and, if they do initiate, discontinue it much earlier. While reassuring counseling is generally correlated with continuation of breastfeeding, women receiving chronic medications still discontinue breastfeeding earlier. Stressing the clear benefits of breastfeeding and the lack of apparent risk of drugs shown to be safe should be coupled with repeated reassurance to mothers during close follow up of their babies.

With few exceptions, medications used by women postpartum are safe for suckling infants because very small amounts of the drugs get through to the baby.[1] Nursing women are often concerned, however, about their drugs having adverse effects on their infants, and this leads them to discontinue breastfeeding. We found that the less reassuring physicians were about the compatibility of a drug with breastfeeding, the higher the incidence of stopping breastfeeding.[2] The Motherisk Program is receiving increasing numbers of queries about maternal medications during breastfeeding. As part of follow up of mothers receiving chronic drug therapy, babies should be routinely monitored for signs or symptoms of ill effects.

In a Motherisk study, we showed that epileptic women tended to breastfeed at about half the rate of control subjects and to breastfeed for a substantially shorter period.[2] We have shown similar trends in women treated for hyperthyroidism with propylthiouracil[3] and women treated with 5-aminoacetylsalicylic acid for inflammatory bowel disease.[4] We have also shown that continuation of breastfeeding is correlated with the cumulative amount of reassuring counseling advice women receive from health professionals.[4]

DURATION OF BREASTFEEDING

In another study, we looked prospectively and closely at a group of nursing women who were reassured by Motherisk that the drugs they wanted to use were safe. We divided the women into two groups according to whether they eventually did or did not take our advice to continue the drugs and compared the duration of breastfeeding in the two groups.[5]

We enrolled 88 women who were exclusively breastfeeding infants younger than 6 months. Follow-up interviews were conducted every 4 weeks until the women completely stopped breastfeeding or the infants reached 7 months of age.

Group 1 consisted of 69 women who reported that they continued the drugs after the counseling session; group 2 consisted of the remaining 19 who said they decided not to start therapy throughout the study period. The women in group 2 gave the following reasons for not continuing their medications: 18 (95%) "did not need" the drugs; and 1 (5%) was "told not to take the drug by a physician." Of the 18 women who did not need the medications, three still expressed concern about the toxicity of their medications for their breast-fed infants. The two groups were not significantly different in demographic characteristics (Table 3–1).

Of the 69 women in group 1, 36 (52%) introduced formula supplementation before infants reached 6 months of age; of 19 in group 2, four (21%) did so ($P = 0.03$). In group 1, 22 (32%) women completely

TABLE 3–1.
DEMOGRAPHIC CHARACTERISTICS OF 88 NURSING WOMEN WHO
DID OR DID NOT CONTINUE DRUG THERAPY POSTPARTUM

Characteristic	Continued Drug Therapy, $N = 69$	Discontinued Drug Therapy, $N = 19$	P Value
Mother's age (years)	32.2 ± 4.5	31.4 ± 4.5	0.48*
Parity			0.19†
1	36	6	
2	22	7	
≥3	11	6	
Infants age (day)			0.27†
≤60	42	10	
61–120	19	4	
121–180	8.6	5	
Mean age of all the infants	0.9 ± 45.6	67.3 ± 52.8	
Mother's education (years)			0.48‡
9–13	11	5	
≥14	58	14	
Marital status			0.86‡
Married	64	17	
Single	2	1	
Cohabiting	3	1	
Family income ($)			0.14‡
<40,000	11	6	
40,000–79,999	33	5	
≥80,000	18	7	
No response	6	1	
Mother employed (years/n)	19/50	10/9	0.07‡

*Unpaired t test.
†Contingency table analysis (df2).
‡χ^2 test with continuity correction (df1).

stopped breastfeeding by the time their infants were 6 months of age (four women stopped breastfeeding by 3 months); only one (5%) of the 19 women in group 2 did so ($P = 0.04$).

Women who took drugs (group 1) tended to introduce formula earlier than those who did not (group 2) ($P < 0.001$). Hence, women in group 2 tended to breastfeed longer than those in group 1 ($P < 0.03$).

Overall, it appears that women who do not continue drug therapy breastfeed exclusively for longer periods and continue breastfeeding longer overall. A similar trend was observed in the analysis of disease-matched subgroups.

Our results indicate that maternal drug therapy during breastfeeding is a risk factor for relatively early introduction of formula supplementation and cessation of breastfeeding. Cumulative reassuring advice is associated with a better chance of continuation of breastfeeding; negative advice is associated with early termination of breastfeeding.[3] Women who chose to continue drug therapy in the study[5] (group 1) did not comply with breastfeeding as well as those who decided not to take drugs. Because we could not ethically have a control group who were not counseled positively about the safety of drugs, we cannot measure the effect of counseling.

BOTTOM LINE

What is the practical point for those who need to counsel nursing mothers taking chronic medication? You might succeed in reassuring them enough to initiate breastfeeding while receiving drug therapy, but be aware that eventually they may discontinue breastfeeding earlier than if they had not taken the drugs. Special efforts should be made to encourage these women not to stop breastfeeding through repeated reassuring counseling.

REFERENCES

1. Taddio A, Ito S. Drugs in breastfeeding. In: Koren G, ed. *Maternal-Fetal Toxicology: A Clinician's Guide.* 2nd ed. New York, NY: Marcel Dekker; 1994.
2. Ito S, Moretti M, Chu M, et al. Initiation and duration of breastfeeding in women receiving antiepileptic drugs. *Am J Obstet Gynecol* 1995;172: 881–886.

3. Lee A, Ito S, Moretti M, et al. The safety of propylthiouracil during breast-feeding; current medical practice [abstract]. *Clin Invest Med* 1998; 514(Suppl 21):S14.

4. Moretti M, Spiczynski Y, Hashemi G, et al. Prospective follow up of infants exposed to 5-aminosalicylic acid containing drugs through maternal milk [abstract]. *Clin Invest Med* 1998;514(Suppl 21):S16.

5. Moretti M, Ito S, Koren G. Initiation and compliance with breastfeeding in women receiving medications. *Pediatr Perinat Drug Ther* (in press).

CHAPTER 4

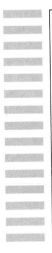

CONTINUING DRUG THERAPY WHILE BREASTFEEDING: COMMON MISCONCEPTIONS OF PHYSICIANS

Gideon Koren, MD, FRCPC
Myla Moretti, MSc
Shinya Ito, MD

QUESTION

Is there any way to predict whether a drug taken by a mother is safe for a suckling baby, or is it just trial and error? One of my patients is receiving lithium for manic depression. She wishes to breastfeed, but clinically there is no way she can discontinue the drug. My sources say the drug is incompatible with breastfeeding.

Answer

The amount of drug available to a baby through breastmilk is estimated as the percentage of maternal dose per kilogram ingested by the baby. Because the infant's clearance rate of many drugs is slower than the adult's, however, the true level of the drug circulating in the infant's blood might be much higher. Because lithium can be measured in plasma, it is prudent to measure it in milk and to estimate the "baby dose." If a baby shows any adverse effects, lithium levels should be measured in its blood.

Many women need drug therapy during the postpartum period to treat chronic or acute medical conditions. Mothers are naturally concerned about the potential risk to their suckling infants from drugs introduced through milk. Hence, it is crucial to identify methods that accurately define the safety or risk of such exposures, because every year scores of new drugs are introduced to the market.

For many years, the ratio between drug concentrations in maternal milk (m) and plasma (p) was used to estimate how much was getting through to a baby. The higher the m/p ratio, the higher concentrations were available to a baby, people assumed. This approach, however, was too simplistic from a pharmacokinetic viewpoint, because a drug's clearance rate from a baby's body is as important as the amount of drug offered to the baby.

Several years ago, the Motherisk team developed a new concept, the exposure index (EI), which incorporated both the m/p ratio and the clearance rate of the drug.[1] The formula is

$$EI = \frac{100 \times m/p \text{ ratio}}{\text{clearance (mL/kg/min)}}$$

The EI, in simple terms, is the percentage of maternal dose per kilogram available to the baby. This equation implies that, even if a drug appears at higher concentrations in milk than in maternal plasma, the clearance rate of the drug will define its safety. Experimental data show that this new concept better estimates the risk to the baby than the old m/p ratio.[1]

In the case of lithium, which has a high m/p ratio, the EI is unsafely high in many infants, but, due to individual (faster) renal clearance rates, is quite low in many others. In several recent cases, we allowed women receiving lithium, who attended Motherisk, to breastfeed, provided lithium levels were measured in breastmilk or neonatal blood. In other cases, such measurements proved the drug unsafe. We concluded that therapeutic drug monitoring could help ascertain whether breastfeeding was safe for women receiving drugs for which there are readily available methods of measurements.

Another relatively common misconception among physicians is in their approach to breastfeeding for women who drink alcohol or smoke cigarettes. While common sense dictates not drinking while breastfeeding, many women are chemically dependent and are unable to discontinue drinking. Advising them not to breastfeed ignores the increased morbidity and mortality among formula-fed babies. Dr. Jack Newman eloquently stated the case: "Those using drugs are also at the risk on many levels for increased infant morbidity and mortality. It is when the socioeconomic situation is the worst that breastfeeding has the greatest benefit."[2]

REFERENCES

1. Ito S, Koren G. A novel index for expressing exposure of infants to drugs in breastmilk. *Br J Clin Pharmacol* 1994;38:99–102.
2. Newman J. Drugs in breastfeeding. *Motherisk Newsletter* 1995;4:4.

PART II

DRUG SAFETY— A TO Z

CHAPTER 5

DRUG SAFETY— A TO Z

Gideon Koren, MD, FRCPC

	Pregnancy risk-benefit	Breastfeeding
Abacavir antiviral	No apparent malformations risk in relatively small series. Untreated maternal HIV may lead to transmission to fetus/newborn. See page 312	human immunodeficiency virus (HIV) may transfer to suckling baby from milk.
Abciximab antiplatelet	Large molecule (Fab antibody) that does not appear to cross the placenta. Only case reports with no apparent malformation risk.	No reported cases, but large molecule not likely to appear in milk. Advantages of breast-feeding should be considered.
Acarbose antidiabetic	Limited systemic absorption from the gut. No apparent malformation risk in limited numbers.	No reported cases, but very limited absorption into mother's circulation. Similar limited absorption is expected if baby is exposed to some of it in milk. Advantages of breastfeeding should be considered.

(Continued)

	Pregnancy risk-benefit	Breastfeeding
Acebutolol beta-blocker, anti-hypertensive	Has been used in hypertension in pregnancy. No apparent malformation risk based on small numbers. No apparent risk of growth retardation.	In small numbers— most babies okay, but there are descriptions of neonatal hypotensions and bradycardia. Proposed monitoring: heart rate. Advantages of breastfeeding should be considered.
Acetaminophen analgesic-antipyretic	Compatible; no apparent malformation risk based on large numbers. Drug of choice for pain in pregnancy.	Compatible
Acetazolamide diuretic	No apparent malformation risk based on small numbers.	No apparent neonatal risks based on small numbers. Advantages of breastfeeding should be considered.
Acetohexamide oral-hyperglycemic	No data on first trimester use. Near term- may cause neonatal hypoglycemia. Insulin and glyburide do not appear to cross the placenta.	No human reports. Proposed monitoring: neonatal hypoglycemia. Advantages of breastfeeding should be considered.
n-Acetyl cysteine mucolytic, antidote	No apparent malformation risk in several reported series. Acetaminophen overdose is a leading cause of suicide attempt in pregnancy and NAC may be critical to maternal health.	No reported cases. Women unlikely to breastfeed when taking NAC. Advantages of breastfeeding should be considered.

(Continued)

	Pregnancy risk-benefit	Breastfeeding
Acitretin severe psoriasis/ keratosis	A potent human teratogen. Limb, craniofacial malformations (retinoid embryopathy). See pages 245, 251	No human data.
Acyclovir antiviral	No apparent malformation risk based on a large registry. Drug of choice to protect newborn from maternal herpes virus. Effective against varicella pneumonia which may be life threatening in late pregnancy. May protect the fetus from varicella infection which is teratogenic (2 to 3% risk).	No apparent neonatal risk in few cases. Much higher doses are used relatively safely in neonates treated for neonatal herpes infection. Advantages of breastfeeding should be considered.
Adalimumab immunoglobulin	No human data, but the large molecule unlikely to cross the human placenta in appreciable amounts.	No human data. Not likely to cross to milk and even if yes—will not be absorbed by suckling baby. Advantages of breastfeeding should be considered.
Adapalene topical cream	No human data to draw conclusion. Very low systemic absorption.	No human data. Very low absorption expected into maternal blood/milk. Advantages of breastfeeding should be considered.
Adefovir anti-HIV	No apparent malformation risk based on small numbers. Untreated maternal HIV or hepatitis B increase risk and fetal infection. See page 312	No human reports. HIV crosses from milk to suckling baby.

23

(Continued)

	Pregnancy risk-benefit	Breastfeeding
Adenosine antiarrhythmic	No apparent malformation risk based on small number of cases. Untreated maternal dysrhythmia can be serious/life threatening.	No human reports. Used as intravenous (IV) injection, and has short elimination half-life. Proposed monitoring: heart rate. Advantages of breastfeeding should be considered.
Albendazole antihelmintic	No apparent systemic absorption. Unclear risk based on small number of cases. No fetal risk in second trimester in controlled studies.	No human data. Due to minimal absorption—probably no neonatal risk. Advantages of breastfeeding should be considered.
Albuterol beta-sympathomimetic	No apparent malformations risk based on large registry. May cause transient fetal/neonatal tachycardia. Used in tocolytic and for asthma. Untreated maternal asthma may bear risks to mother and fetus. Decreases risk of neonatal respiratory distress syndrome.	No human data. Probably safe when inhaled by mother for asthma. Advantages of breastfeeding should be considered.
Alendronate biphosphonate	No apparent malformation risk in few published cases. No apparent teratogenic risk in animals. Very limited systemic absorption, but released from bone over years.	No human data, but limited systemic absorption into maternal blood/milk and similarly if ingested in milk— very limited absorption into baby. Advantages of breastfeeding should be considered.

(Continued)

	Pregnancy risk-benefit	Breastfeeding
Alfentanil opioid analgesic	No first trimester exposure has been reported, but opioid narcotics are not teratogenic in animals or humans. When used for surgery near term—neonates/central nervous system (CNS) depression is possible and should be treated.	Amounts excreted into human milk—small. The drug not expected to be absorbed through the gastrointestinal tract (GiT) of the suckling infant. Proposed monitoring: CNS depression. Advantages of breastfeeding should be considered.
Allopurinol xanthine oxidase inhibitor	No apparent malformation risk based on small number of cases.	No apparent neonatal risks based on small numbers. Advantages of breastfeeding should be considered.
Almotriptan antimigraine	No human reports. Much larger, favorable experience with sumatriptan, drug of the same class.	No human data. Advantages of breastfeeding should be considered.
Alosetron antidiarrheal antiemetic	No human data. Larger, favorable experience with another member of this class, ondansetron for morning sickness.	No human data. Advantages of breastfeeding should be considered.
Alphaprodine opioid analgesic	No first trimester reports. At term, may cause neonatal CNS depression or withdrawal that need to be followed up (f/u) and treated.	No human data. Unlikely to be absorbed significantly by the suckling infant. Proposed monitoring: CNS depression.

(Continued)

	Pregnancy risk-benefit	Breastfeeding
Alprazolam benzodiazepine	No apparent malformation risk based on a large registry. Neonatal withdrawal should be anticipated and treated when used near term. Maternal addiction must be considered with its attendant risks during pregnancy and parenthood. See page 184	Small amounts excreted into milk. Proposed monitoring: CNS depression and/or withdrawal.
Alteplase thrombolytic (t-PA)	No apparent malformation risk based on a few cases. Very short half-life (5 minutes) A large molecule unlikely to cross the placenta. Treatment of maternal risks of thrombosis may be critical.	No human data. Even if reaches the milk—it is not likely to be absorbed in the baby's gut. Advantages of breastfeeding should be considered.
Amantadine, antiviral, anti-parkinsonian	Small numbers suggested increased malformation risks, which did not reach statistical significance.	No human reports. The low amounts secreted into milk probably preclude neonatal risks. Advantages of breastfeeding should be considered.
Ambenonium cholinergic	No apparent malformation risk based on few cases. Consider maternal morbidity when the drug is used for myasthenia gravis.	No human data. Being a polar molecule, probably small amounts in milk. Advantages of breastfeeding should be considered.
Amikacin aminoglycoside	No human safety data in first trimester. Unlikely to cause malformations or hearing loss. Systemic maternal infection needs to be treated.	Small amounts in milk. No apparent neonatal risk has been reported.

(Continued)

	Pregnancy risk-benefit	Breastfeeding
Amiloride diuretic	No apparent malformation risk based on small numbers. If used for maternal hypertension-there are diuretics with more safety data (e.g., thiazides).	No human reports. Proposed monitoring: urine output, electrolytes. Advantages of breastfeeding should be considered.
Amino-glutethimide anticonvulsant	No apparent malformation risk based on small number of cases. There are antiepileptics with much larger favorable safety data (carbamazepine, lamotrigine).	No human data. Advantages of breastfeeding should be considered.
Aminopterin anticancer	Causes a specific pattern of malformation. CNS, cranial, limb, lip-palate. See page 150	Breastfed infant should not be exposed to anticancer drugs through milk.
para-Aminosalicylic acid anti-TB	No apparent malformation risk based on small numbers except for one study. Maternal TB must be treated. Other anti-TB drugs have more safety data (e.g., isoniazid)	No human safety data. Amounts in milk are low and probably safe. Advantages of breastfeeding should be considered.
Amiodarone	No apparent malformation risk based on small numbers of cases. Neonatal thyroid function should be monitored. The risk of the maternal condition (typical—serious dysrhythmia) must be considered.	Large amounts excreted into milk, which contains large amounts of iodine.

(Continued)

	Pregnancy risk-benefit	Breastfeeding
Amitriptyline antidepressant	No apparent malformation risk based on controlled studies. When used at term—infants may experience a withdrawal syndrome, and should be monitored closely, un/subtreated maternal depression can have serious risk. See pages 290, 293, 297	No apparent neonatal risk based on small numbers. Advantages of breastfeeding should be considered.
Amlodipine calcium channel blocker	No human reports. Other drugs of same class (e.g., nifedipine) have more safety data.	No human reports. Proposed monitoring: blood pressure. Advantages of breastfeeding should be considered.
Ammonium chloride expectorant, urinary acidifie	No apparent malformation risk in a relatively small number of reports.	No human data. Advantages of breastfeeding should be considered.
Amobarbital sedative hypnotic	Limited human data on first trimester use is contradictory (both negative and positive reports of malformation risk).	No human data. Proposed monitoring: CNS depression.
Amoxapine antidepressant	No sufficient human data. Other agents of the same class do not exhibit apparent malformation risk. Neonate may exhibit poor adaptation syndrome. See pages 290, 293, 297	No apparent neonatal toxicity in small numbers of cases. Advantages of breastfeeding should be considered.

(Continued)

	Pregnancy risk-benefit	Breastfeeding
Amoxicillin penicillin antibiotic	No apparent malformation risk based on large numbers.	No apparent neonatal risk based on available data. Proposed monitoring: diarrhea due to potential change in gut flora. Advantages of breastfeeding should be considered.
Amphetamine CNS stimulant	No apparent malformation risk based on epidemiological studies. If taken as part of addiction, consider various medical and psychosocial risks of addiction. Should not be used for weight control in pregnancy. Very rare justified indications (e.g., severe narcolepsy).	No apparent neonatal risk in very limited data. Proposed monitoring: CNS status.
Amphotericin antifungal	No apparent malformation risk in small numbers of cases. If mother needs treatment for systemic fungal infection—the risk of not treating her is serious.	No human data. Advantages of breastfeeding should be considered.
Ampicillin penicillin antibiotic	No apparent malformation risk based on large numbers.	No apparent neonatal risk based on large numbers. Proposed monitoring: diarrhea due to potential change in gut flora.

(Continued)

	Pregnancy risk-benefit	Breastfeeding
Amprenavir anti-HIV	No apparent malformation risk based on small numbers. Optimal treatment of maternal HIV infection is critical for both mother and fetus. Agents with more human experience include zidovudine, nevirapine. See page 312	Women positive to HIV should not breastfeed due to milk transmission of the virus.
Amrinone inotrope	No first trimester safety data exist. Treatment of congestive heart failure may be critical for maternal and fetal health.	No human data exist.
Amyl nitrate vasodilator	No apparent malformation risk based on very small numbers.	No human data. Proposed monitoring: blood pressure perfusion.
Anagrelide antiplatelet	No apparent malformation risk based on very small numbers. May be critical to treat maternal disorder.	No human data.
Anakinra immunomod-ulator	No human data. The large molecular size (17,000) consistent with minimal/no transfer. Severity of maternal condition and need for therapy must be considered.	No human data. Probably limited/no penetrance to milk, and even if yes, limited/no oral absorption by baby.
Anisindione anticoagulant	No apparent malformation risk based on small numbers. May be critical to treat maternal condition.	No human data.
Anthralin antipsoriatic	No human data.	No human data.

(Continued)

	Pregnancy risk-benefit	Breastfeeding
Antipyrine analgesic antipyretic	No apparent malformation risk in very small numbers.	No human data.
Antithrombin III	A naturally occurring agent. Use for preeclampsia in second to third trimesters not associated with apparent fetal risks.	No human data.
Argatroban (antithrombin)	No human data. May be critical to treat maternal condition.	No human data.
Aripiprazole antipsychotic	No human reports. It may be critical to treat maternal schizophrenia. There are medications with larger human experience (e.g., haldol, celanzepine, risperidone).	No human data. Proposed monitoring: CNS status.
Asparaginase anticancer	Anticancer drugs inhibit cell division and may cause malformation in first trimester. See page 150	Breastfed infant should not be exposed to cancer drugs through milk.
Aspartame sweetener	No apparent malformation risk when used by healthy women. Should be used cautiously in women with phenylketonuria (PKU).	No apparent neonatal risk except in cases of PKU.
Acetylsalicylic acid NSAID	No apparent evidence of overall malformation risk. Apparent increased risk (twofold) for gastroschisis. In late pregnancy—may cause premature closure of fetal ductus arteriosus. See pages 154, 242	No apparent neonatal risks. Proposed monitoring: bleeding. Advantages of breastfeeding should be considered.

(Continued)

	Pregnancy risk-benefit	Breastfeeding
Astemizole antihistamine	No apparent malformation risk based on small numbers. No apparent malformation risk for antihistamines as a group based on large numbers. See page 161	No apparent neonatal risk based on small numbers.
Atazanavir anti-HIV	No apparent malformation risk based on small numbers. It is critical to treat effectively maternal HIV infection for maternal and fetal health. See page 312	HIV crosses to breast milk and may infect the baby.
Atenolol beta-blocker	No apparent malformation risk in a few studies. Association with intrauterine growth retardation. Neonate may exhibit beta-blockade.	There are cases of extensive transfer to breast—milk and potential toxicity. Proposed monitoring: blood pressure, heart rate.
Atomoxetine attention deficit disorder	No apparent malformation risk based on very few cases.	No human data.
Atorvastatin statin	Statins may interfere with fetal cholesterol synthesis. Spontaneous FDA reports on statins suggests increased teratogenic risk (CNS, limbs). A small prospective study does not support it. See page 159	No human data. May interfere with cholesterol synthesis in the neonate.
Atovaquone antiprotozoal	No apparent fetal risk in third trimester when used for malaria.	No human data. Advantages of breastfeeding should be considered.

(Continued)

	Pregnancy risk-benefit	Breastfeeding
Atracurium muscle relaxant	No data on first trimester. Has been used safely in second to third trimester to paralyze fetus before various fetal procedures.	No human data.
Atropine parasym-patholytic	No apparent malformation risk in small numbers available.	No human data.
Azatadine antihistamine	No apparent malformation risk in small numbers (for azatadine), and in very large numbers to all antihistamine as a class. See page 161	No human data. Advantages of breastfeeding should be considered.
Azathioprine immuno-suppressant	No apparent malformation risk based on relatively small numbers. Important to treat organ transplant effectively.	No apparent neonatal risk based on small numbers. Advantages of breastfeeding should be considered.
Azelastine antihistamine	No human reports. Antihistamines as a class have not been associated with teratogenicity. This compound, used topically is probably safe. See page 161	No human data. Probably very low/ none of the topically administered drug will reach the milk. Advantages of breastfeeding should be considered.
Azithromycin antibiotic	No apparent malformation risks in small numbers available.	No apparent neonatal risk in a few cases. Advantages of breastfeeding should be considered.

(Continued)

	Pregnancy risk-benefit	Breastfeeding
Baclofen muscle relaxant	No apparent malformation risk based on few cases available.	Limited human experience, very small weight-adjusted dose in milk. Advantages of breastfeeding should be considered.
Balsalazide agent for anti-inflammatory bowel disease	No human data, but it is metabolized to 5-aminosalicylic acid (mesalamine) for which there is no apparent teratogenic risk based on small controlled studies.	No human data. No apparent evidence of neonatal risk with mesalamine. Advantages of breastfeeding should be considered.
Beclomethasone corticosteroid	No apparent malformation risk in small numbers available when inhaled. Because of its low bioavailability—very low systemic concentrations produced. See pages 154, 236	No human data. Very likely that minimal/no amounts reached the milk from maternal inhalation.
Belladonna parasym-patholytic	A controlled 1960s study of 554 cases suggested increased malformation risk (respiratory, hypospadias, eye and ear). No other study is available as the drug is rarely used today.	No human data.
Benazepril Angiolensin-converting enzyme (ACE) inhibitor anti-hypertensive	No apparent malformation risk in first trimester, based on small available numbers. In third trimester can cause fetal renal failure oligohydramnios and hypocalciuria. See pages 198, 204	No human data.

(Continued)

	Pregnancy risk-benefit	Breastfeeding
Benzphetamine sympathomimetic anorexiant	Should not be used in pregnancy. No reports in human pregnancy.	No human data.
Benztropine parasympatholytic	No apparent malformation risk in small available numbers. As a class—larger numbers of atropine derivatives did not exhibit malformation risk.	No human data.
Beta carotene vitamin	No apparent malformation risk in few available cases. Being a precursor of the teratogenic vitamin A, women should not use it at daily levels above the recommended (400 IU per day). See pages 218	No neonatal safety data available. Vitamin A is a natural constituent of human milk.
Betamethasone corticosteroid	When used in late pregnancy to induce fetal lung maturation—large reports of increased risk of periventricular leucomalacia and brain damage. See pages 154, 236	No human data.
Betaxolol beta-blocker antihypertensive	No apparent fetal risk based on small studies. There are beta-blockers with much larger favorable human experience (e.g., labetalol).	No apparent neonatal risk based on small numbers. Proposed monitoring: neonatal bradycardia, hypotension, poor perfusion.
Bethanechol parasympathomimetic	No apparent malformation risk based on small available numbers.	No human data.

(Continued)

	Pregnancy risk-benefit	Breastfeeding
Bexarotene antineoplastic retinoid	Being a retinoid and anticancer contraindicated in pregnancy. See page 150	No human data.
Bismuth subsalicylate antidiarrheal	No apparent malformation risk based on small numbers.	No human data. Due to low systemic bioavailability of bismuth—minimal/no excretion into milk is expected. Salicylate will appear in milk (see aspirin). Advantages of breastfeeding should be considered.
Bisoprolol beta-blocker antihypertensive	No human data. Beta-blocker exposure has been associated with intrauterine growth retardation. There are beta-blockers with large experience in pregnancy (labetalol, atenolol)	No human data. Proposed monitoring: beta-blockade. Advantages of breastfeeding should be considered.
Bivalirudin thrombin inhibitor	Large molecular weight (mw 2180) and very short half-life (25 minutes)—probably marginal/no fetal exposure. No human report. Complications of clotting pathology may be life threatening.	No human data. Advantages of breastfeeding should be considered.

(*Continued*)

	Pregnancy risk-benefit	Breastfeeding
Bleomycin anticancer	Contraindicated in first trimester as it exerts its effects through inhibition of DNA synthesis. A few cases of second to third trimester exposure with normal babies. May cause neonatal neutropenia, anemia or thrombocytopenia. See page 150	Breastfed infant should not be exposed to cancer drugs through milk.
Blue Cohosh herb—labor induction	There are case reports of uterine tetany and birth asphyxia. Preparations are not standardized and checked for content of active ingredients. See page 194	No data. Advantages of breastfeeding should be considered.
Bosentan vasodilator for pulmonary artery hypertension	No human data. In animals—defects in head, mouth, face, blood vessels, shown also with other endothelin receptor antagonists. Maternal condition may needs to be treated.	No human data. Advantages of breastfeeding should be considered.
Botulinum Toxin A for motor nerve paralysis	No evidence of apparent fetal risk in several pregnancies with botulinum infection. When used as local injection, the toxin is likely not entering the systemic circulation.	No human data. Advantages of breastfeeding should be considered.

(Continued)

	Pregnancy risk-benefit	Breastfeeding
Bromide sedative	No apparent malformation risk based on large prospective study. At terms—neonatal CNS depression may occur. See page 184	Rash and sedation have been described in breastfed infants.
Bromocriptine treatment of hyperpro- lactinemia	No apparent malformation risk in large numbers, including apparent normal development.	Inhibits lactation by decreasing prolactin levels.
Brompheniramine antihistamine	One prospective study suggested increased malformation risks, based on 65 cases. Another prospective study did not confirm it. There are better studied H_1 blockers (e.g., diphenhydramine, chlorpheniramine). As a group, H_1 blockers have not shown teratogenic risk based on large numbers. See page 161	Limited data does not suggest increased neonatal risk. Proposed monitoring: sedation. Advantages of breastfeeding should be considered.
Buclizine antihistamine antiemetic	No apparent risk of malformations in a small study. There are antiemetics with substantially more safety data (e.g., diclectin, doxylamine). As a group— antihistamines have not been shown to be teratogenic.	No human data. Advantages of breastfeeding should be considered.

(Continued)

	Pregnancy risk-benefit	Breastfeeding
Budesonide Inhaled corticosteroid	No apparent risk of malformations in relatively large studies, in distinction from systemic corticosteroids. See page 236	No human data. Only small amounts enter maternal blood, and hence appearance in milk and then in infants blood is unlikely. Advantages of breastfeeding should be considered.
Bumetanide diuretic	No apparent malformation risk based on a small study. There are diuretics with much more data in pregnancy (e.g., thiasides, furosemide).	No human data. may suppress milk production. Advantages of breastfeeding should be considered.
Buprenorphine mixed agonist-antagonist opioid	No studies of use during embryogenesis. In small numbers: Use in later pregnancy (toward birth) uneventful. May cause CNS depression or neonatal withdrawal.	In one controlled study—less weight gain while breast-feeding with the drug as compared to bupivaccine. Proposed monitoring: CNS depression.
Bupropion antidepressant, smoking inhibition	No apparent malformation risk in several studies. See pages 290, 293, 297	No apparent neonatal risk when breastfeeding with the drug.
Buspirone anxiolytic	No apparent malformation risk in small studies. Neonatal withdrawal may occur. See page 184	No human data. There are sedative hypnotics with human data (e.g., benzodiazepines). Proposed monitoring: sedation.

(Continued)

	Pregnancy risk-benefit	Breastfeeding
Busulfan antineoplastic	May cause malformations by inhibiting cell division in first trimester. See page 150	No human studies. The baby should not be exposed to anticancer drugs through milk.
Butalbital sedative, tension headache	No apparent malformation risk in several studies. Neonatal withdrawal may occur. See page 184	No human studies. Proposed monitoring: CNS depression.
Butaperazine tranquilizer	No human data. Phenothiazines have not been associated with increased malformation risk.	No human data. Proposed monitoring: CNS depression.
Butoconazole antifungal	No apparent malformation risk in first trimester in one study. No apparent fetal risk when used in second to third trimesters.	No human data. Advantages of breastfeeding should be considered.
Butorphanol mixed agonist-antagonist opioid	No data in first trimester. May cause neonatal CNS depression and/or withdrawal syndrome.	No apparent neonatal risk in one case. Levels in milk are low. Proposed monitoring: CNS depression.
Cabergoline antihyper-prolactinemia	The drug of choice to induce pregnancy in hyperprolactinemia. No apparent fetal risk based on several studies.	Suppresses milk production.
Caffeine	No apparent malformation risk. Daily dose above 150 mg associated with increased miscarriage rate. See page 164	No apparent neonatal risk. Advantages of breastfeeding should be considered.

(Continued)

	Pregnancy risk-benefit	Breastfeeding
Calcitonin hormone	No human data. Probably does not cross the placenta (large peptide).	No human safety data. Probably does not cross into milk. Advantages of breastfeeding should be considered.
Camphor topical anesthetic	No apparent malformation risk when applied topically, based on a relatively large study.	No human study. Topical application will likely not result in appreciable milk levels.
Candesartan cilexetil antihypertensive	Angiotensin II receptor antagonists, similar to ACE inhibitor, may cause fetal-neonatal renal failure, with oligohydramnios, hypocalvaria. Should be avoided in second and third trimesters. See pages 198, 204	No human reports. Advantages of breastfeeding should be considered. Proposed monitoring: urine output, blood pressure.
Capreomycin antituber-culosis	No human data. There are anti-TB drugs with safety data (e.g., INH, rifampin).	No human data.
Captopril antihyper-tensive	ACE inhibitors do not appear to increase malformation risk in first trimester. In second and third trimesters they can cause fetal-neonatal renal failure, oligohydramnion and hypocalvaria. Neonatal death from renal failure may occur. See pages 198, 204	No apparent neonatal risk in small series. Proposed monitoring: urine output, blood pressure.

(*Continued*)

	Pregnancy risk-benefit	Breastfeeding
Carbachol ophthalmic cholinergic	No human data. Systemic levels probably negligible after ophthalmic use.	No human data. Milk levels probably negligible after ophthalmic use. Advantages of breastfeeding should be considered.
Carbamazepine antiepileptic	Risk of about 1% for neural tube defects (NTD). Detailed ultrasound and alfafeto proteins should rule out NTD. Widely used for epilepsy in pregnancy. Vitamin K supplementation (10 to 20 mg per day) 4 weeks before expected delivery.	No apparent neonatal risk while breastfeeding based on small numbers. Advantages of breastfeeding should be considered.
Carbarsone amebicide	Although no reports in human pregnancy were located, the drug contains arsenic which can be neurotoxic to the fetus.	No human data.
Carbenicillin penicillin	No apparent malformation risk based on small numbers.	No human data. No apparent neonatal risk with other penicillins. Proposed monitoring: diarrhea due to potential change in gut flora.
Carbidopa antiparkinson	No apparent malformation risk based on small numbers.	No human data.
Carboplatin anticancer	Inhibits cell division and therefore can cause malformations in first trimester. See page 150	Women should not breastfeed while on anticancer drugs.

(Continued)

	Pregnancy risk-benefit	Breastfeeding
Carisoprodol muscle relaxant	No apparent malformation risk based on small numbers.	No data on neonatal risk. High milk levels have been measured.
Carmustine (BCNU) Anticancer	Inhibits cell division and therefore can cause malformations in first trimester. See page 150	Women should not breastfeed while on anticancer drugs.
Carphenazine tranquilizer	No human data. There are other phenothizines with large safety data (e.g., haldol).	No human data. Proposed monitoring: CNS depression.
Carteolol beta-blocker	No human studies. Beta-blockers are associated with intrauterine growth retardation. There are beta-blockers with large experience (e.g., labetalol).	No human data. Advantages of breastfeeding should be considered. Proposed monitoring: blood pressure.
Carvedilol alpha and beta-blocker	No human studies. There are beta-blockers with large experience (e.g., labetalol).	No human data. Advantages of breastfeeding should be considered.
Casanthranol laxative	No apparent malformation risk in one study.	No human data. Advantages of breastfeeding should be considered.
Cascara sagrada laxative	No apparent malformation risk in one study.	Limited human data. Proposed monitoring: diarrhea due to potential change in gut flora.
Caspofungin antifungal	No human data.	No human data. High molecular weight (1213) and high protein binding preclude high milk levels.

(Continued)

	Pregnancy risk-benefit	Breastfeeding
Cefaclor cephalosporin	No apparent malformation risk based on relatively large numbers. No apparent malformation risk for cephalosporins as a group.	No apparent neonatal risks based on small numbers. Proposed monitoring: diarrhea due to potential change in gut flora.
Cefadroxil cephalosporin	No apparent malformation risk based on relatively small numbers. No apparent malformation risk for cephalosporins as a group.	No apparent neonatal risks based on small numbers. Proposed monitoring: diarrhea due to potential change in gut flora.
Cefamandole	No apparent malformation risk based on relatively small numbers. No apparent malformation risk for cephalosporins as a group.	No apparent neonatal risks based on small numbers. Proposed monitoring: diarrhea due to potential change in gut flora.
Cefatrizine cephalosporin	No human data. No apparent malformation risk for cephalosporins as a class.	No human safety data. Low milk levels. Advantages of breastfeeding should be considered. Proposed monitoring: diarrhea due to potential change in gut flora.
Cefazolin cephalosporin	No apparent malformation risk based on small numbers. No apparent malformation risk for cephalosporins as a group.	No human safety outcome data. Low milk levels. Advantages of breastfeeding should be considered. Proposed monitoring: diarrhea due to potential change in gut flora.

(Continued)

	Pregnancy risk-benefit	Breastfeeding
Cefdinir cephalosporin	No human reports. No apparent malformation risk for cephalosporins as a group.	No human data. Advantages of breastfeeding should be considered. Proposed monitoring: diarrhea due to potential change in gut flora.
Cefditoren cephalosporin	No human reports. No apparent malformation risk for cephalosporins as a group.	No human data. Low milk levels. Advantages of breastfeeding should be considered. Proposed monitoring: diarrhea due to potential change in gut flora.
Cefepime cephalosporin	No human data. No apparent malformation risk for cephalosporins as a group.	No human safety data. Low milk levels. Advantages of breastfeeding should be considered. Proposed monitoring: diarrhea due to potential change in gut flora.
Cefixime cephalosporin	No apparent malformation risk based on small numbers. No apparent malformation risk for cephalosporin as a class.	No human reports. Advantages of breastfeeding should be considered. Proposed monitoring: diarrhea due to potential change in gut flora.
Cefmetazole cephalosporin	No human data. No apparent malformation risk for cephalosporins as a class.	No human data. Advantages of breastfeeding should be considered. Proposed monitoring: diarrhea due to potential change in gut flora.

(*Continued*)

	Pregnancy risk-benefit	Breastfeeding
Cefonicid cephalosporin	No human data. No apparent malformation risk for cephalosporins as a class.	No human safety data. Low milk levels. Proposed monitoring: diarrhea due to potential change in gut flora.
Cefoperazone cephalosporin	No apparent malformation risk in relatively small numbers. No apparent malformation risk for cephalosporin as a class.	No human safety data. Low milk levels. Proposed monitoring: diarrhea due to potential change in gut flora.
Cefotaxime cephalosporin	No apparent malformation risk in relatively small numbers. No apparent malformation risk for cephalosporin as a class.	No human safety data. Low milk levels. Proposed monitoring: diarrhea due to potential change in gut flora.
Cefotetan cephalosporin	No human safety data. No apparent malformation risk of cephalosporins as a class in humans. No apparent malformation risk for cephalosporin as a class.	No safety data in humans. Low levels in milk. Proposed monitoring: diarrhea due to potential change in gut flora.
Cefoxitin cephalosporin	No human safety data. No apparent malformation risk for cephalosporin as a class.	No safety data in humans. Low levels in milk. Proposed monitoring: diarrhea due to potential change in gut flora.
Cefrozil cephalosporin	No human safety data. No apparent malformation risk for cephalosporin as a class.	No safety data in humans. Low levels in milk. Proposed monitoring: diarrhea due to potential change in gut flora.

(Continued)

	Pregnancy risk-benefit	Breastfeeding
Ceftazidime cephalosporin	No human safety data. No apparent malformation risk for cephalosporin as a class.	No safety data in humans. Low levels in milk. Proposed monitoring: diarrhea due to potential change in gut flora.
Ceftizoxime cephalosporin	No human safety data reported. No apparent malformation risk of cephalosporin as a class.	No safety data in humans. Low levels in milk. Proposed monitoring: diarrhea due to potential change in gut flora.
Ceftriaxone cephalosporin	No apparent malformation risk in limited numbers. No apparent malformation risk for cephalosporin as a class.	No safety data in humans. Low levels in milk. Proposed monitoring: diarrhea due to potential change in gut flora.
Cefuroxime cephalosporin	No apparent malformation risk in limited numbers. No apparent malformation risk for cephalosporin as a class.	No safety data in neonates. Low milk levels. Proposed monitoring: diarrhea due to potential change in gut flora.
Celecoxib Nonsteroidal anti-inflammatory	No human reports on malformations. No complications at term. May cause preterm closure of ductus arteriosus. See pages 154, 242	Low milk levels. Advantages of breastfeeding should be considered.
Celiprolol beta-blocker	No human data. There are beta-blocker with large safety data (e.g., labetalol, propranolol). Beta-blockers are associated with intrauterine growth retardation.	No human data. Advantages of breastfeeding should be considered. Proposed monitoring: blood pressure, heart rate.

(Continued)

	Pregnancy risk-benefit	Breastfeeding
Cephalexin cephalosporin	No apparent malformation risk based on several studies. No apparent malformation risk for cephalosporins as a class in humans.	No apparent neonatal risk. Advantages of breastfeeding should be considered. Proposed monitoring: diarrhea due to potential change in gut flora.
Cephalothin cephalosporin	No human reports. No apparent malformation risk for cephalosporins as a class in humans.	Low milk concentrations. No neonatal safety data. Advantages of breastfeeding should be considered. Proposed monitoring: diarrhea due to potential change in gut flora.
Cephopirin cephalosporin	No human data. No apparent malformation risk for cephalosporins as a class in humans.	Low milk levels. No neonatal safety data. Advantages of breastfeeding should be considered. Proposed monitoring: diarrhea due to potential change in gut flora.
Cephradine cephalosporin	No apparent malformation risk in relatively small numbers. No apparent malformation risk for cephalosporins as a class.	Low milk levels. No neonatal safety data. Advantages of breastfeeding should be considered. Proposed monitoring: diarrhea due to potential change in gut flora.

(Continued)

	Pregnancy risk-benefit	Breastfeeding
Cerivastatin antilipemic	Inhibition of cholesterol synthesis may potentially affect fetal development. FDA case reports suggest limb and CNS malformation. Small Prospective studies do not show apparent malformation risk. See page 159	Should not be used as it may affect cholesterol synthesis in baby.
Cetirazine nonsedating antihistamine	No apparent malformation risk based on small numbers. No apparent malformation risk for H_1 blockers as a class, based on large numbers. See page 161	No human data. As a class, H_1 blockers do not cause an apparent neonatal risk based on large numbers. Advantages of breastfeeding should be considered.
Cevimeline cholinergic	No human data.	No human data. Advantages of breastfeeding should be considered. Proposed monitoring: cholinergic signs.
Chenodiol gall stone solubilizer	No human data. Observed neonatal hepatotoxicity in some animals.	No human data.
Chloral hydrate sedative hypnotic	No apparent malformation risk in small series.	Drowsiness in a breastfed baby was described. Advantages of breastfeeding should be considered. Proposed monitoring: CNS depression.

(Continued)

	Pregnancy risk-benefit	Breastfeeding
Chlorambucil anticancer	Anticancer drugs can inhibit cell division and may adversely affect fetal development in first trimester. See page 150	Breastfeeding should not take place with anticancer drugs.
Chloramphenicol antibiotic	No apparent malformation risk in limited numbers.	Low milk levels. No data on neonatal safety. Advantages of breastfeeding should be considered. Proposed monitoring: diarrhea due to potential change in gut flora.
Chlordiazepoxide sedative	Both association and lack of association with malformations were described. Neonatal withdrawal may occur.	No human data. Proposed monitoring: sedative effects. Advantages of breastfeeding should be considered.
Chlorhexidine topical anti-infective	No data on first trimester use, but systemic levels with topical use are negligible.	No human data, but systemic levels with topical use are negligible. Advantages of breastfeeding should be considered.
Chloroquine antimalaria, anticollagen disease	No apparent malformation risk based on several small series. See page 168	Low levels in milk. No neonatal safety data. Advantages of breastfeeding should be considered.
Chlorothiazide diuretic	No apparent malformation risk in several limited studies.	No apparent neonatal risk. Low milk levels. Proposed monitoring: urine output.

(Continued)

	Pregnancy risk-benefit	Breastfeeding
Chlorpheniramine antihistamine	No apparent malformation risk in large numbers. No apparent malformation risk for H_1 blockers as a class. See page 161	No apparent neonatal risk. Advantages of breastfeeding should be considered.
Chlorpromazine tranquilizer	No apparent malformation risk based on relatively large numbers. Extrapyramidal syndrome if used at term.	May cause neonatal drowsiness and sedation. Advantages of breastfeeding should be considered.
Chlorpropamide oral hypoglycemia	No apparent malformation risk based on small numbers. Can cause neonatal hypoglycemia when taken in late pregnancy.	No human data. Proposed monitoring: neonatal hypoglycemia.
Chlorprothixene tranquilizer	No human data.	No human data. Proposed monitoring: CNS depression.
Chlorthalidone diuretic	No human data. There are diuretics with fetal safety data (e.g., thiazides).	No human data. Advantages of breastfeeding should be considered. Proposed monitoring: urine output.
Chlorzoxazone muscle relaxant	No apparent malformation risk based on limited data.	No human data.
Cholestyramine antilipidemic	Not absorbed in the gut. No apparent malformation risk based on relatively large data. Binds fat soluble vitamins, so mother's vitamin status must be monitored carefully. See page 159	Not absorbed hence cannot appear in milk. Advantages of breastfeeding should be considered.

(Continued)

	Pregnancy risk-benefit	Breastfeeding
Ciclopirox topical antifungal	No human reports, but systemic absorption through the skin is minimal.	No human data. Unlikely to appear in milk. Advantages of breastfeeding should be considered.
Cidofovir antiviral	No human data. There are antivirals for HIV and cytomegalovirus (CMV) with fetal safety data (zidovudine). Treating effectively is critical for maternal and fetal outcome. See page 312	Women with HIV should not breastfeed due to viral transfer through milk.
Cigarette smoking	Associated with increased rates of miscarriage, stillbirth, prematurity, intrauterine growth retardation, sudden infant death syndrome. See page 171	Small amounts of smoke constituents pass to milk. The advantages of breastfeeding over-weight potential neonatal (but unproven) risks.
Ciguatoxin fish neurotoxin	No apparent malformation risk based on small numbers. Apparent fetal toxicity was described at term.	A case of neonatal toxicity was described. Baby should not be breastfed when mother experiences toxicity.
Cilostazol antiplatelet agent	No human data. Treating mother may be critical.	No human data. Advantages of breastfeeding should be considered.
Cimetidine H_2 blocker	No apparent malformation risk based on relatively large data. See page 281	No neonatal safety. Advantages of breastfeeding should be considered. Proposed monitoring: GiT symptoms.

(*Continued*)

	Pregnancy risk-benefit	Breastfeeding
Cinoxacin quinolone	No human data. There are quinolones with fetal safety data (e.g., ciprofloxacin).	No human data. Advantages of breastfeeding must be considered. Suggested monitoring: diarrhea due to potential change in gut flora.
Ciprofloxacin quinolone antibiotic	No apparent malformation risk based on relatively large data.	No apparent fetal risk in limited data. Advantages of breastfeeding should be considered. Proposed monitoring: diarrhea due to potential change in gut fora.
Cisapride gastrointestinal prokinetic	No apparent malformation risk based on several studies. See page 281	Limited human data showing very low levels in the suckling neonate. Proposed monitoring: gastrointestinal symptom.
Cisplatin	The drug is capable of causing malformations by inhibiting cell division in first trimester. See page 150	Newborns should not be exposed to anticancer drugs through milk.
Citalopram antidepressant	No apparent malformation risks based on several controlled studies. When taken at term, 10% to 30% of babies may experience self-limited poor neonatal adaptation syndrome. See pages 290, 293, 297	No apparent neonatal risk based on a small number of cases. Proposed monitoring: sleeparousal, irritability, breathing. Advantages of breastfeeding should be considered.

(Continued)

	Pregnancy risk-benefit	Breastfeeding
Clarithromycin antibiotic	No apparent malformation risk based on several studies.	Low levels in breast-milk Proposed monitoring: diarrhea due to possible change in gut flora. Advantages of breastfeeding should be considered.
Clavulanic acid anti-infective	No apparent malformation risk based on a large study.	No human data. Proposed monitoring: diarrhea due to possible change in gut flora. Advantages of breastfeeding should be considered.
Clemastine antihistamine	No apparent malformation risk based on a large study. Antihistamines as a group—no increased teratogenic risk. See page 161	Limited human data. Watch for neonatal sedativeness, drowsiness. Advantages of breastfeeding should be considered.
Clindamycin antibiotic	No apparent malformation risk based on a large study.	Low milk concentrations. Proposed monitoring: diarrhea due to change in gut flora. Advantages of breastfeeding should be considered.
Clofazimine antilepra	No apparent malformation risk based on small numbers.	Watch for skin pigmentation in the baby. Advantages of breastfeeding should be considered.
Clofibrate antilipemic	No human data. See page 159	No human data.

(Continued)

	Pregnancy risk-benefit	Breastfeeding
Clomiphene fertility	No apparent increased malformation risk in small studies, but case reports of neural tube defects.	No human data.
Clomipramine tricyclic antidepressant	No apparent teratogenic risk based on relatively small numbers. No apparent malformation risk for tricyclic antidepressants as a group. At term—poor neonatal adaptation syndrome may occur. See pages 290, 293, 297	No apparent neonatal risk in small numbers. Proposed monitoring: signs of poor adaptation syndrome. Advantages of breastfeeding should be considered.
Clonazepam antiepileptic	No apparent malformation risk in several studies. No apparent malformation risk for benzodiazepines, except for unclear risk of oral cleft (see Lorazepam). Neonatal toxicity (CNS depression) or withdrawal may occur. See page 184	Limited human data. Proposed monitoring: CNS depression. Advantages of breastfeeding should be considered.
Clonidine antihyper-tensive	No apparent malformation risk based on small numbers.	No apparent neonatal toxicity in a small number of cases. Proposed monitoring: neonatal blood. pressure and perfusion.
Clopidogrel antiplatelet	No apparent malformation risk in single cases. There are antiplatelets with wider record of fetal safety (e.g., aspirin).	No human data. Advantages of breastfeeding should be considered. Proposed monitoring: platelets, bleeding.

(*Continued*)

	Pregnancy risk-benefit	Breastfeeding
Clorazepate sedative	No human data. Benzodiazepines as a class have not been shown to increase teratogenic risk except for unclear association with oral cleft. Neonatal CNS depression or withdrawal can occur. See page 184	No human data. Proposed monitoring: CNS depression and neonatal withdrawal.
Clotrimazole antifungal	No apparent malformation risk based on small numbers. Topical use not likely to cause clinically significant systemic exposure.	No human data. Milk exposure unlikely with topical use. Advantages of breastfeeding should be considered.
Cloxacillin penicillin	No apparent malformation risk in small numbers. Penicillin as a class— not associated with malformation risk.	No human data. Penicillins excreted at low levels in milk. Proposed monitoring: diarrhea due to potential change in gut flora. Advantages of breastfeeding should be considered.
Clozapine antipsychotic	No apparent malformation risk based on small numbers.	No human data. Proposed monitoring: CNS effects. Advantages of breastfeeding should be considered.
Cocaine stimulant	Associated with low birth weight, intrauterine growth retardation, prematurity, stillbirth, placental abruption.	No apparent neonatal risk based small numbers. Proposed monitoring: CNS excitation, measuring cocaine-benzoylecgonine in milk.

(Continued)

	Pregnancy risk-benefit	Breastfeeding
Codeine opioid analgesic,	No apparent malformation risk in small numbers. Neonate may experience CNS depression or withdrawal.	Limited human data. May cause CNS depression. If mother is ultra rapid CYP2D6 metabolizer, baby may be toxic. Proposed monitoring: CNS depression, opioid toxicity.
Colchicine antigout antifamilial Mediterranean fever	No apparent malformation risk based on small numbers. Several babies with Down's, possibly due to the drug's mutagenic effect. See page 174	No apparent neonatal risk in small number of cases. Advantages of breastfeeding should be considered.
Colesevelam antilipemic	This polymer is not absorbed through the gut. May affect absorption of fat soluble vitamins (D, E, K, A). See page 159	Lack of systemic absorption renders the drug safe for the baby.
Colestipol antilipemic	This resin is not absorbed through the gut. May affect absorption of lipid soluble vitamins (D, E, K, A). See page 159	Lack of systemic absorption renders the drug safe for the suckling baby.
Colistimethate antibiotic	No human data.	Small amounts in milk. No neonatal safety data. Proposed monitoring: diarrhea due to potential change in gut flora.

(*Continued*)

	Pregnancy risk-benefit	Breastfeeding
Coumadins anticoagulants	First trimester use may cause the *fetal warfarin syndrome* in up to 10% of fetuses exposed in first trimester: cartilage and bone defects, nasal hypoplasia, stippled epiphyses, eye defects, CNS effects in second trimester: Dandy-Walker malformations, mental retardation. See page 179	No apparent neonatal risk in a small number of cases. Phenindione resulted in bleeding in a suckling infant. Proposed monitoring: bleeding.
Cromolyn sodium antiasthma	No apparent malformation risk in several large studies.	No human data. Advantages of breastfeeding should be considered. Minimal levels are expected due to low systemic levels (Hale).
Cyclacillin penicillin	Very limited human data. Penicillins as a class do not exhibit apparent malformation risk based on large numbers.	No human reports. Penicillins are excreted in low levels into milk. Proposed monitoring: diarrhea due to potential change in gut flora. Advantages of breastfeeding should be considered.
Cyclamate sweetener	No human data.	No human data. Advantages of breastfeeding should be considered.
Cyclazocine opioid antagonist	No human data.	No human data. Advantages of breastfeeding should be considered.

(Continued)

	Pregnancy risk-benefit	Breastfeeding
Cyclizine antihistamine	No apparent teratogenic risk in small numbers. Antihistamines as a class do not exhibit apparent malformation risks based on large numbers. See page 161	No data available Proposed monitoring: CNS depression. Advantages of breastfeeding should be considered.
Cyclobenzaprine muscle relaxant	No apparent malformation risk based on a large study.	No human data. Advantages of breastfeeding should be considered. Proposed monitoring: CNS changes.
Cyclophos-phamide anticancer	Cancer drugs inhibit cell division and may cause malformations in first trimester. See page 150	The infant should not be exposed to cancer drugs through breast milk.
Cycloserine antituberculosis	No apparent malformation risk based on very few cases. There are anti-TB drugs with much larger fetal safety data (e.g., izoniazide, rifampicin)	No apparent neonatal risk based on small numbers. Advantages of breastfeeding should be considered.
Cyclosporine immuno-suppressant	No apparent malformation risk or developmental delays based on relatively large numbers.	No apparent neonatal risk based on small numbers.
Cyproheptadine antihistamine, antiserotonin	No apparent malformation risk in one relatively large study.	No human studies. Can lower prolactin and inhibit milk production.
Cytarabine anticancer	Cancer drugs inhibit cell division and may cause anticancer malformations in first trimester. See page 150	Infants should not be exposed to cancer drugs through breast milk.

(*Continued*)

	Pregnancy risk-benefit	Breastfeeding
Dacarbazine anticancer	Cancer drugs inhibit cell division and may cause malformations in first trimester.	Infants should not be exposed to cancer drugs through breast milk.
Dactinomycin anticancer	Cancer drugs inhibit cell division and may cause malformations in first trimester. See page 150	Infants should not be exposed to cancer drugs through breast milk.
Dalteparin anticoagulant	Low molecular weight heparins do not cross the human placenta. No apparent malformation risk based on relatively large number of cases. See page 208	Does not transfer to milk.
Danaparoid anticoagulant	Low molecular weight heparins do not cross the placenta. No apparent malformation risk based on small numbers. See page 208	Does not transfer to milk.
Danazol androgen	May affect female fetal genitalia and virilization based on small numbers.	The suckling infant should not be exposed to androgens through breast milk.
Dantrolene muscle relaxant	No first trimester experience. Late pregnancy exposure for maternal malignant hyperthermia—no apparent fetal risk in small numbers.	No human experience. Due to short half-life not expected to appear in milk 2 days after maternal treatment.

(*Continued*)

	Pregnancy risk-benefit	Breastfeeding
Dapsone antilepra, antimalarial	No apparent malformation risk based on small numbers. See page 168	Limited human data. No report of neonatal risk. Advantages of breastfeeding should be considered. Proposed monitoring: diarrhea due to potential changes in gut flora.
Darbepoetin hematopoietic	Due to large molecular weight—unlikely to cross the placenta (mw 37,000).	Unlikely to transfer into milk due to large molecular size.
Daunorubicin anticancer	Cancer cells inhibits cell division and may cause malformations in first trimester. See page 150	The suckling infant should not be exposed to cancer drugs through breast milk.
Deferoxamine iron chelator	No apparent malformation risk based on small numbers.	Not absorbed well orally, and hence, even if appears in milk— unlikely to be absorbed by the infant's gut. Advantages of breastfeeding should be considered.
Delavirdine anti-HIV	No apparent malformation risk based on small numbers. See page 312	HIV may cross to the baby through breast milk.
Demecarium cholinergic	No human experience.	No human experience.
Desflurane anesthetic gas	Anesthetic gases have been associated with miscarriage risk among exposed health professionals. No apparent fetal risk when used at term. See page 231	No human data. Low to unmeasurable milk levels 24 hours after anesthetic use.

(Continued)

	Pregnancy risk-benefit	Breastfeeding
Desipramine tricyclic antidepressant	No apparent malformation risks based on limited numbers. Tricyclics as a class do not exhibit apparent malformation risk. Poor neonatal adaptation syndrome may occur. See pages 290, 293, 297	No apparent neonatal toxicity in small numbers. Proposed monitoring: CNS changes.
Dexamethasone corticosteroid	Systemic exposure to corticosteroids has been associated with two- to threefold increased risk of oral cleft CNS? See pages 154, 236	No human data. Advantages of breastfeeding should be considered.
Dextromethorphan antitussive	No apparent malformation risk based on several large studies.	No neonatal safety data. Advantages of breastfeeding should be considered.
Diatrizoate diagnostics contrast media	Contains high levels of organic iodine. Intraamniotic injection: No apparent effect on fetal thyroid based on small series, but elevated TSH in another series.	No milk levels in a single case. Proposed monitoring: thyroid function.
Diazepam sedative	No apparent increased malformation risk based on several studies. Possible, but unclear association with oral cleft. Baby may show sedative effects or withdrawal. See page 184	No apparent neonatal risk based on limited numbers. Proposed monitoring: sedation and other CNS effects. Advantages of breastfeeding should be considered.

(Continued)

	Pregnancy risk-benefit	Breastfeeding
Diazoxide antihypertensive	No apparent malformation risk based on small numbers. May cause fetal bradycardia after rapid use. May cause uterine relaxation. Should be given cautiously in severe hypertension. Proposed neonatal monitoring: blood pressure, hyperglycemia.	No human data.
Dichlorphenamide diuretic	No human data. There are diuretics with fetal data. (thiazide, furosomide).	No human data.
Diclectin antinauseant	Safe based on a large number of controlled studies. See page 190	No apparent neonatal risk based on small series.
Diclofenac nonsteroidal anti-inflammatory	No apparent malformation risk based on several large studies. May cause tocolysis and premature closure of ductus arteriosus. See pages 154, 242	No human data. Advantages of breastfeeding should be considered.
Dicloxacillin penicillin	No apparent malformation risk based on small numbers. For penicillin as a group—no apparent malformation risk based on large numbers.	No human reports. No apparent neonatal risks for penicillin. Proposed monitoring: diarrhea due to potential change in gut flora.
Dicyclomine parasympatholytic	No apparent malformation risk based on large numbers.	Several case reports of neonatal apnea. These cases could not prove causation.

(Continued)

	Pregnancy risk-benefit	Breastfeeding
Didanosine anti-HIV	No apparent malformation risks based on small numbers. Maternal therapy is needed to improve health and prevent vertical transmission of HIV. See page 312	HIV may transfer to milk.
Dienestrol estrogen	No apparent malformation risk based on large numbers.	No human data.
Diethylpropion anorexiant	No apparent congenital risk based on over 1000 women.	No neonatal safety data.
Diethylstilbestrol estrogen	Causes vaginal carcinoma in some adolescents exposed in utero (1:1000). In some men exposed in utero: testicular, penile and sperm anomalies.	No human data.
Diflunisal nonsteroidal anti-inflammatory	No apparent malformation risk based on several available studies. NSAIDs may cause premature closure of ductus arteriosus in late pregnancy. See pages 154, 242	No neonatal safety data available. Advantages of breastfeeding should be considered.
Digoxin, digitoxin cardiac glycosides	No apparent malformation risk in small numbers. Drug of choice for fetal dysrhythmias.	No neonatal safety data available. The amounts available in milk are small. Advantages of breastfeeding should be considered. Proposed neonatal monitoring: heart rate.

(Continued)

	Pregnancy risk-benefit	Breastfeeding
Digoxin immune FAB	No apparent malformation risk based on case reports. A protein, unlikely to cross the placenta in clinically relevant amounts.	No data.
Dihydrocodeine opioid	No reports during embryogenesis. Used mostly during labor. Baby may exhibit opioid effects (CNS depression), or withdrawal.	No apparent neonatal risk in most babies. If mother is ultra rapid CYP2D6 metabolizer—baby may be toxic from larger amounts of morphine produced. Proposed monitoring: signs of opioid toxicity.
Diltiazem calcium channel blocker	No apparent malformation risk based on small numbers.	No apparent neonatal risk based on several case reports. Advantages of breastfeeding should be considered.
Dimenhydrinate antihistamine	No apparent malformation risk based on several studies. No apparent malformation risk with antihistamines based on very large numbers. See page 161	No human data. Antihistamines may cause neonatal sedation. Proposed monitoring: CNS depression. Advantages of breastfeeding should be considered.
Dimercaprol chelator	No apparent malformation risk based on small numbers of case reports. Most cases occurred after first trimester.	No human data.

(*Continued*)

	Pregnancy risk-benefit	Breastfeeding
Dimethindene antihistamine	No apparent malformation risk based on small numbers. No apparent malformation risk for antihistamines as a class based on very large numbers. See page 161	No human data. Antihistamines may cause neonatal sedation. Proposed monitoring: CNS depression. Advantages of breastfeeding should be considered.
Diphenhydramine antihistamine	No apparent malformation risk based on large numbers.	No human safety data. Antihistamines may cause neonatal sedation. Proposed monitoring: CNS depression. Advantages of breastfeeding should be considered.
Diphenoxylate antidiarrheal opioid	No apparent malformation risk based on small numbers.	No human data. Opioids may cause CNS depression.
Dipyridamole antiplatelets	No apparent malformation risk based on small numbers.	No human safety data. Proposed monitoring: bleeding phenomena. Advantages of breastfeeding should be considered.
Disopyramide antiarrhythmic	No apparent malformation risk based on small numbers.	No apparent neonatal risk based on small numbers. Proposed monitoring: heart rate and rhythm. Advantages of breastfeeding should be considered.
Disulfiram antialcohol abuse	No apparent malformation risk based on small numbers.	No human data.

(*Continued*)

	Pregnancy risk-benefit	Breastfeeding
Dobutamine sympath-omimetic	No human data. There are sympathomimetic agents with more safety data (e.g., dopamine, norepinephrine).	No human data. Proposed monitoring: heart rate, blood pressure. Advantages of breastfeeding should be considered.
Docusate sodium laxative	No apparent malformation risk based on small numbers.	No apparent neonatal risk based on small numbers. Advantages of breastfeeding should be considered.
Dofetilide antiarrhythmic	No human data. There are fetal safety data on a variety of antiarrhythmics (e.g., digoxin, quinidine, verapamil, amiodarone).	No human data. Proposed monitoring: heart rhythm. Advantages of breastfeeding should be considered.
Dolasetron antiemetic	No human data. There are 5HT3 antagonists with fetal safety data (e.g., ondansetrone).	No human data.
Domperidone antiemetic-lactation stimulant	No human data during embryogenesis.	Increases milk production when used for this cause in many countries. No apparent neonatal risk.
Donepezil cholinesterase inhibitor	Used mostly in Alzheimer, hence no human data in pregnancy.	No human data.
Dopamine sympath-omimetic	Mostly used in late pregnancy for eclampsia. No apparent fetal risk based on small numbers.	No human data. Advantages of breastfeeding should be considered.

(Continued)

	Pregnancy risk-benefit	Breastfeeding
Dothiepin tricyclic antide-pressants	No apparent risk of malformations based on small numbers. Tricyclics have not been associated with malformations or neurocognitive effects based on relatively large numbers. Poor neonatal adaptation syndrome may occur. See pages 290, 293, 297	No apparent neonatal risk, for tricyclics, including neurocognitive development based on small numbers. Advantages of breastfeeding must be considered.
Doxapram respiratory stimulant	No human data. There are respiratory stimulants with fetal safety data (e.g., caffeine, theophylline).	No human data. Advantages of breastfeeding should be considered. Proposed monitoring: CNS stimulation.
Doxepin tricyclic antidepressant	No apparent malformation risk based on small numbers. No apparent malformation risk or neurocognitive effects for tricyclic anti-depressants based on relatively large numbers. Poor neonatal adaptation syndrome may occur. See pages 290, 293, 297	Several case reports of CNS depression and hypotonia.
Doxorubicin anticancer	May affect cell division and hence may induce malformations in first trimester. No apparent risk when used in late pregnancy, based on small numbers.	Suckling infants should not be exposed to cancer drugs through breast milk.

(Continued)

	Pregnancy risk-benefit	Breastfeeding
Doxylamine antihistamine antiemetic	No apparent malformation risk based on very large numbers. See page 161	No apparent neonatal risk in small number. Antihistamine in breast milk may cause CNS depression. Proposed monitoring: CNS status. Advantages of breastfeeding should be considered.
Droperidol tranquilizer antiemetic	No apparent malformation risk based on small numbers.	No human data.
Drotrecogin alfa thrombolytic	No apparent malformation risk based on small numbers. It is doubtful whether this protein crosses the placenta.	No human data. Very unlikely to cross into milk.
Echinacea herb	No apparent malformation risk based on small numbers. See page 194	No human data. Advantages of breastfeeding should be considered.
Econazole antifungal	Available only topically. Minimal systemic absorption. No evidence of apparent fetal adverse events based on small numbers.	No human data. Systemic and milk absorption probably marginal. Advantages of breastfeeding should be considered.
Ecstasy (MDMA) stimulant	No apparent malformation risk based on small numbers.	No human data.
Ethylenedi-aminetetra-acetic acid (EDTA) antidote	No apparent malformation risk based on small number of cases.	No human data. If it is given for maternal lead poisoning—milk may introduce large amounts of lead.

(Continued)

	Pregnancy risk-benefit	Breastfeeding
Edrophonium cholinergic	No human data.	No human data.
Efavirenz anti-HIV	No apparent malformation risk based on small numbers. See page 312	HIV may transfer from milk to suckling infant.
Electric current	Hand to foot current that crosses the womb may cause fetal death.	Irrelevant.
Eletriptan antimigraine	No human reports. There are other drugs of the same class with relatively large fetal safety data (sumatriptan).	No neonatal safety data available. Advantages of breastfeeding should be considered.
Emtricitabine anti-HIV	No apparent malformation risk based on a few cases See page 312	HIV may infect the infant through breast milk.
Enalapril antihyper-tensive	No apparent malformation risk based on small numbers. Can cause fetal renal shutdown, hypocalvaria, oligohydramnion and neonatal death when used in late pregnancy. See pages 198, 204	No neonatal safety data available. Advantages of breastfeeding should be considered. Proposed monitoring: neonatal blood pressure, perfusion.
Encanide antiarrhythmic	No human safety data during embryogenesis. Used safety to treat fetal dysrhythmia.	No human data.
Enflurane general anesthetic	No safety data during embryogenesis (first trimester). No apparent risk when used for caesarian section. Increased risk of miscarriage among health professional working in ORs.	No human data.

(Continued)

	Pregnancy risk-benefit	Breastfeeding
Enfuvirtide HIV antiviral	No fetal safety data. There are HIV antivirals with fetal safety data. See page 312	HIV may infect suckling infants through breast milk.
Enoxacin quinolone antibacterial	No apparent malformation risk based on small numbers. Quinolones as a class do not appear to increase malformation risk based on relatively large numbers.	No human reports. Proposed monitoring: diarrhea due to potential changes in gut flora.
Enoxaparin low molecular heparin	The molecule does not appear to cross the placenta. See page 208	The molecule too large to cross into milk, and even if it does— it won't likely be absorbed in the infant's gut.
Entocapone antiparkin- sonian	No human data.	No human data.
Ephedrine sympath- omimetic	No apparent malformation risk based on one relatively large series.	A single case report with adverse events (irritability, sleep problem). Proposed monitoring: blood pressure, heart rate, CNS stimulation.
Epinephrine sympath- omimetic	No apparent malformation risk based on small numbers.	No human data.
Epirubicin anticancer	Anticancer drugs may cause malformation in first trimester by inhibiting cell growth and division. See page 150	The suckling baby should not be exposed to cancer drugs.

(Continued)

	Pregnancy risk-benefit	Breastfeeding
Epoprostenol, a vasodilator prostaglandin	Very short half-life in blood (6 minutes). Almost no reports of use in first trimester. No apparent fetal risk in late pregnancy.	No human reports. Its rapid degradation precludes large milk exposure. Advantages of breastfeeding should be considered.
Epoetin alfa erythropoietin	This large peptide appears to cross the human placenta. No apparent malformation risk based on small numbers.	No human data. Probably marginal passage into milk. Unlikely to be absorbed by the neonatal gut.
Eprosartan antihyper-tensive	No human data in one to two trimesters. In third trimester this angiotensin II receptor antagonists may cause fetal oliguria-anuria, hypocalvaria and oligohydramnion similar to ACE inhibitors.	No human data.
Eptifibatide antiplatelet	No human data.	No human data. Even if small amounts of this peptid appear in milk—unlikely to be absorbed intact by baby.
Ergotamine antimigraine	Small and infrequent doses do not appear to be linked to fetotoxicity or teratogenicity. Larger doses or frequent use may cause fetal toxicity or teratogenicity due to maternal/fetal vascular disruption (Briggs). Ergot derivatives can cause uterine contractions.	A 1934 study reported ergalism in babies (vomiting, diarrhea, convulsions). The drug may suppress lactation.

(Continued)

	Pregnancy risk-benefit	Breastfeeding
Ertapenem antibiotic	No human data. No evidence of increased malformation risk with other beta lactam antibiotics. (penicillins, cephalosporins).	No human data. Proposed monitoring: diarrhea due to change in gut flora. Advantages of breastfeeding should be considered.
Erythromycin antibiotic	No apparent malformation risk based on large numbers.	No apparent increased neonatal risk. Proposed monitoring: diarrhea due to change in gut flora. Advantages of breastfeeding should be considered.
Esmolol beta-blocker	No human data on use in first trimester. No apparent fetal risk in late pregnancy based on a few cases.	No human data. Proposed monitoring: neonatal blood pressure and heart rate. Advantages of breastfeeding should be considered.
Estazolam hypnotic	No human data. At term, benzodiazepine may cause CNS depression or withdrawal. See page 184	No human data. Advantages of breastfeeding should be considered. Proposed monitoring: CNS depression.
Estradiol estrogen	No apparent malformation risk based on small studies. Meta-analysis of all oral contraceptives failed to show malformation risk.	No apparent neonatal risk based on small numbers. Advantages of breastfeeding should be considered.
Estrogens	No apparent malformation risk based on meta-analyses.	No apparent neonatal risk based on small numbers. Advantages of breastfeeding should be considered.

(Continued)

	Pregnancy risk-benefit	Breastfeeding
Etanercept immunomod-ulator	No apparent malformation risk based on small numbers.	No human data. The protein is unlikely to appear in milk, and subsequently, unlikely to be absorbed by the suckling infant.
Ethacrynic acid diuretic	No apparent malformation risk based on small numbers.	No human data. Proposed monitoring: diuretic effect in neonate. Advantages of breastfeeding should be considered.
Ethambutol anti-TB	No apparent malformation risk based on small numbers.	No apparent neonatal risk based on small numbers. Advantages of breastfeeding should be considered.
Ethanol alcohol	Can cause the fetal alcohol spectrum disorder (growth retardation, facial anomaly, complex neurobehavioral deficits) in offspring of problem drinker. Women should abstain from alcohol in pregnancy.	Alcohol in milk may adversely affect the baby neurocognitively. See page 212
Ethchlorvynol hypnotic	No apparent malformation risk based on small numbers.	No human data. Proposed monitoring: CNS depression, or withdrawal.
Ethinamate hypnotic	No apparent malformation risk based on small numbers.	No human data. Proposed monitoring: CNS depression or withdrawal.

(Continued)

74

	Pregnancy risk-benefit	Breastfeeding
Ethinyl estradiol estrogen	No apparent malformation risk for oral contraceptives based on meta-analyses.	No apparent neonatal risk based small numbers. Advantages of breastfeeding should be considered.
Ethionamide anti-TB	No apparent malformation risk based on small numbers.	No human data. Advantages of breastfeeding should be considered.
Ethosuximide anticonvulsant	No apparent malformation risk based on small numbers.	No data on neonatal risk. Advantages of breastfeeding should be considered.
Ethotoin anticonvulsant	Very few reports. Hydantoins can cause fetal hydantoin syndrome (see phenytoin).	No human data. Advantages of breastfeeding should be considered.
Etodolac nonsteroidal anti-inflammatory	No human data. NSAIDs do not appear to increase malformation risks in repeated studies. They may cause premature closure of ductus arteriosus in late pregnancy. See pages 154, 242	No human data. No apparent neonatal risk for NSAIDs. Advantages of breastfeeding should be considered.
Etoposide anticancer	Anticancer drugs can inhibit cell division and cause malformations in first trimester. No apparent malformation risk beyond first trimester. See page 150	Suckling infants should not be exposed to cancer drugs through breast milk.
Etretinate retinoid	Retinoid embryopathy includes CNS malformation, face anomalies, cardiac defects. See pages 251, 256	No human data.

75

	Pregnancy risk-benefit	Breastfeeding
Ezetimibe antilipemic	No human data.	No human data.
Famciclovir antiviral	No apparent malformation risk based on small numbers.	No human data.
Famotidine H_2 antihistamine blocker	No apparent malformation risk based on small numbers. No apparent malformation risk for H_2 blockers based on meta-analysis. See page 281	No data on neonatal safety. Advantages of breastfeeding should be considered.
Felbamate antiepileptic	No human data.	No human data on neonatal safety. Advantages of breastfeeding should be considered.
Felodipine calcium channel blocker	No apparent malformation risk for the drug, based on small number. No apparent risk for calcium channel blockers based on small numbers.	No human data. Advantages of breastfeeding should be considered. Proposed monitoring: blood pressure.
Fenfluramine anorexiant	No human data during embryogenesis. No apparent risk after embryogenesis in small numbers.	No human data.
Fenofibrate antilipemic	No human data. Disruption of fetal cholesterol may potentially affect fetal development. See page 159	No human data. Disruption of neonatal cholesterol may potentially affect neonatal development.
Fenoldopam antihypertensive	No human data.	No human data.

(*Continued*)

	Pregnancy risk-benefit	Breastfeeding
Fenoprofen nonsteroidal anti-inflammatory	No apparent malformation risk based on small numbers. No apparent malformation risk for NSAIDs based on large numbers. NSAIDs may cause premature closure of fetal ductus arteriosus in late pregnancy. See pages 154, 242	No data on neonatal safety. No apparent neonatal risk for NSAIDs as a group, based on small numbers. Advantages of breastfeeding should be considered.
Fenoterol beta-sympa-thomimetic	No human data in first trimester. No apparent fetal-neonatal toxicity during labor in small numbers.	No human data. Proposed monitoring: neonatal heart rate, blood pressure. Advantages of breastfeeding should be considered.
Fentanyl opioid	No human data in first trimester. No apparent fetal toxicity later in pregnancy and during birth. Neonatal CNS depression can occur.	No data on neonatal safety. Proposed monitoring: CNS depression.
Fenoxfenadine antihistamine	No apparent malformation risk for the drug based on small numbers. No apparent malformation risk for antihistamines based on large numbers. See page 161	No apparent neonatal risk for antihistamines. Proposed monitoring: CNS depression. Advantages of breastfeeding should be considered.
Filgrastim hematopoietic	Crosses the placenta despite large molecular weight. No apparent malformation risk based on small numbers.	No human data. Even if this large molecule appears in milk—unlikely to be absorbed in baby. Advantages of breastfeeding should be considered.

(Continued)

	Pregnancy risk-benefit	Breastfeeding
Flavoxate antispasmodic (bladder)	No data on first trimester exposure. No apparent fetal toxicity in second to third trimester based on small studies.	No human data. Proposed monitoring: neonatal urinary output.
Flecanide antiarrhythmic	No apparent malformation risk based on small numbers. Effective for fetal tachyarrhythmia.	No data on neonatal safety. Advantages of breastfeeding should be considered. Proposed monitoring: neonatal heart rate.
Fluconazole antifungal	No apparent malformation risk in several cohort studies.	No apparent neonatal risk based on small numbers. Advantages of breastfeeding should be considered.
Flucytosine antifungal	No first trimester data. There are antifungals with some safety data (e.g., ketoconazole, amphotericin).	No human data. Advantages of breastfeeding should be considered.
Flumazenil benzodiazepine antidote	No first trimester data. No apparent fetal toxicity in late pregnancy based on a case report.	No human data.
Flunitrazepam hypnotic	No human data. As a group, benzodiazepines do not appear to increase overall malformation rate. Risk for oral cleft—unclear. May cause neonatal CNS depression or withdrawal. See page 184	No human data. Proposed monitoring: CNS depression.

(*Continued*)

	Pregnancy risk-benefit	Breastfeeding
Fluorouracil anticancer	Cancer drugs inhibit cell division and may cause congenital malformations in the first trimester. See page 150	Breastfed infants should not be exposed to cancer drugs through breast milk.
Fluoxetine antidepressant	No apparent malformation risk or neurocognitive effects based on several cohort studies and meta-analysis. A self-limited neonatal poor adaptation syndrome may occur. Uncontrolled depression increases perinatal risks. See pages 290, 293, 297	No apparent neonatal risk based on small numbers. Decreased weight gain was described but it is not clear whether it is due to the drug or the depression.
Fluoxymesterone androgen	No human data. Androgens may affect sexual development of the female fetus.	No human data.
Fluphenozine tranquilizer	No apparent malformation risk based on small numbers. No apparent malformation risk for phenothiazines based on repeated studies.	No human data on neonatal safety. Proposed monitoring: CNS depression.
Flurazepam hypnotic	No apparent malformation risk based on small numbers. No apparent malformation risk for benzodiazepines based on relatively large numbers. An association with oral cleft was not statistically clear. Neonatal withdrawal syndrome may occur with chronic use.	No human data. Proposed monitoring: CNS depression.

(Continued)

	Pregnancy risk-benefit	Breastfeeding
Flurbiprofen nonsteroidal anti-inflammatory	No human data. No apparent malformation risk for NSAIDs based on repeated studies. NSAIDs may cause premature closure of ductus arteriosus in late pregnancy. See pages 154, 242	No studies on neonatal safety. Very small amounts excreted into milk. Advantages of breastfeeding should be considered.
Fluvastatin antilipemic	No human data. Statins, disrupting cholesterol synthesis, may theoretically affect cholesterol in the fetus (see Lovastatin). See page 159	No human data. Theoretical disruption of cholesterol metabolism in the neonate should be considered and the drug should be avoided until data are available.
Fluvoxamine antidepressant	No apparent malformation risk in repeated studies. No apparent malformation risk for selective serotonin reuptake inhibitor (SSRI) as a group. Poor neonatal adaptation syndrome may occur (irritability, poor feeding, respiratory distress). Untreated maternal depression may increase perinatal risk for mother and fetus. See pages 290, 293, 297	No apparent neonatal risk based on small numbers. Proposed monitoring: CNS. Advantages of breastfeeding should be considered.

(Continued)

	Pregnancy risk-benefit	Breastfeeding
Folic acid vitamin	Optimal use (at least 0.4 mg per day but up to 5 mg per day) decreases risk for neural tube defects, and possibly other malformations (cardiovascular, limb) and pediatric cancer (neuroblastoma). See pages 218, 221	No apparent neonatal risk.
Fomepizole methanol and ethylene glycol antidote	No human data.	No human data.
Fondaparinux anticoagulant	Large molecule used in deep vein thrombosis (DVT) prophylaxis. Does not appear to cross the placenta. Maternal DVT should be treated.	No human data. Unlikely that, even if appears in milk, will be absorbed intact by the infant.
Fosamprenavir anti-HIV	No apparent malformation risk based on very small numbers. Maternal HIV must be treated for both maternal and fetal well being. See page 312	HIV may transfer from milk to suckling infant.
Foscarnet antiviral	No human data in first trimester.	No human data.
Fosfomycin antibiotic	No apparent malformation risk based on small numbers.	No human data. Proposed monitoring: diarrhea due to potential change in gut flora. Advantages of breastfeeding should be considered.

(Continued)

	Pregnancy risk-benefit	Breastfeeding
Frovatriptan antimigraine	No human reports. There is relatively wide fetal safety data on sumatriptan.	No human data.
Furosemide diuretic	No apparent malformation risk based on relatively small numbers. In late pregnancy: diuretics may prevent normal plasma volume expansion.	No data on neonatal safety. Proposed monitoring: urine output, dehydration.
Gabapentin antiepileptic	No apparent malformation risk based on small numbers.	No human data. Advantages of breastfeeding should be considered.
Gadopentetate contrast diagnostic	No human data.	Excreted in very small amounts into milk, manifold lower than the safe IV dose given to neonates.
Ganciclovir antiviral	No apparent malformation risk based on a few case reports.	No human data. Advantages of breastfeeding should be considered.
Gadolinium contrast media	No apparent malformation risk based on small studies. See page 224	No human data. Advantages of breastfeeding should be considered.
Garlic herb	Appears to be safe as food flavoring. No data on high dose in pregnancy. See page 194	No apparent neonatal risk. Advantages of breastfeeding should be considered.
Gatifloxacin quinolone	No human data. There are quinolones with relatively large fetal safety data (e.g., ciprofloxacin)	No human data. Proposed monitoring: diarrhea, due to potential change in gut flora. Advantages of breastfeeding should be considered.

(Continued)

	Pregnancy risk-benefit	Breastfeeding
Gemfibrozil antilipemic	No apparent malformation risk based on small numbers. See page 159	No human data.
Gemifloxacin quinolone	No human data. There are quinolones with relatively large fetal safety data (e.g., ciprofloxacin)	No human data. Proposed monitoring: diarrhea, due to potential changes in gut flora. Advantages of breastfeeding should be considered.
Gentamicin antibiotic	No apparent teratogenic risk based on small numbers.	No apparent neonatal toxicity. Proposed monitoring: diarrhea, due to potential change in gut flora. Advantages of breastfeeding should be considered.
Ginger herb	No apparent malformation risk based on repeated studies. See page 194	No human studies. Advantages of breastfeeding should be considered.
Ginkgo biloba herb	No human data. See page 194	No human reports. Advantages of breastfeeding should be considered.
Ginseng herb	No apparent malformation risk based on small numbers. See page 194	No human data. Advantages of breastfeeding should be considered.
Glimepiride oral hypoglycemic	No human data. There are oral hypoglycemics with large fetal data (e.g., glyburide).	No human data. Proposed monitoring: glucose levels.

(Continued)

	Pregnancy risk-benefit	Breastfeeding
Glipizide oral hypoglycemic	No apparent malformation risk based on small numbers. There are oral hypoglycemics with larger fetal data (e.g., glyburide).	No human data. Proposed monitoring: glucose levels.
Glyburide oral hypoglycemic	Does not appear in fetal circulation, due to high protein binding, short half-life and active transporters effluxing it to the maternal circulation. Does not cause neonatal hypoglycemia. No apparent malformation risks when used in first trimester based on small numbers.	Does not appear in measurable levels in milk. No apparent neonatal toxicity based on small numbers. Proposed monitoring: glucose levels. Advantages of breastfeeding should be considered.
Gold antirheumatic	No apparent malformation risk based on small numbers.	A few cases of adverse events in neonates, although cause-and-effect could not be established. Advantages of breastfeeding should be considered.
Granisetron antiemetic	No human data. There are 5HT3 receptor antagonists with fetal safety data (e.g. ondansetron). See page 190	No human data. Advantages of breastfeeding should be considered.
Griseofulvin antifungal	No apparent malformation risk based on small numbers.	No human data. Advantages of breastfeeding should be considered.
Guaifenesin expectorant	No apparent malformation risk based on small numbers.	No human data. Advantages of breastfeeding should be considered.

(Continued)

	Pregnancy risk-benefit	Breastfeeding
Guanabenz antihypertensive	No human data. There are antihypertensives with fetal safety data.	No human data. Proposed monitoring: blood pressure.
Guanadrel antihypertensive	No human data. There are antihypertensive drugs with fetal safety data.	No human data. Proposed monitoring: blood pressure.
Guanethidine antihypertensive	No apparent malformation risk based on small numbers. There are antihypertensive drugs with wider fetal safety data (e.g., labetalol, methyldopa).	No human data. Proposed monitoring: blood pressure. Advantages of breastfeeding should be considered.
Guanfacine antihypertensive	No apparent malformation risk based on small numbers. There are antihypertensive drugs with larger fetal safety data (e.g., labetalol, methyldopa).	No human data. Proposed monitoring: blood pressure. Advantages of breastfeeding should be considered.
Haloperidol tranquilizer, antipsychotic	No apparent malformation risk based on repeated small studies. If used near term observe the infant for possible extrapyramidal symptoms.	Report of decreased cognitive function in a small number of breastfed infants. Proposed monitoring: CNS depression.
Halothane anesthetic gas	No apparent malformation risk based on small numbers. No apparent fetal neonatal risk when used at term occupational exposure may be associated with small risk of miscarriage. See page 231	No neonatal safety data. Proposed monitoring: CNS depression.

(Continued)

	Pregnancy risk-benefit	Breastfeeding
Hemin (hematin) hematopoietic	No apparent malformation risk in case reports.	No human data.
Heparin anticoagulant	Does not cross the placenta. No apparent malformation risk based on small numbers.	Does not cross into milk.
Heroin opioid analgesic	No apparent malformation risk based on small numbers. Neonatal CNS depression and withdrawal can occur.	Can cause CNS depression and neonatal addiction. Proposed monitoring: CNS depression, neonatal withdrawal.
Hexachlorophene topical antiseptic	No apparent malformation risk when used topically in recommended doses, in repeated studies.	No data on neonatal safety. When used on nipples-thorough wash should precede breastfeeding.
Hexoprenaline sympath-omimetic	No data on first trimester use. Although no apparent neonatal risk when used for tocolysis, case reports of maternal and fetal tachycardia described.	No human data. Proposed monitoring: heart rate, blood pressure.
Hydralazine antihyper-tensive	No apparent malformation risk based on small numbers.	No neonatal safety data. Proposed monitoring: blood pressure. Advantages of breastfeeding should be considered.
Hydrocodone opioid analgesic	No apparent malformation risk based on small numbers. Can cause CNS depression and neonatal withdrawal.	No human data. May cause CNS depression. Proposed monitoring: CNS depression and neonatal withdrawal.

(Continued)

	Pregnancy risk-benefit	Breastfeeding
Hydrocortisone corticosteroid	Systemic use in first trimester associated with increased risk or oral cleft. See pages 154, 236	No human reports, but levels in milk are unlikely to be clinically significant. Advantages of breastfeeding should be considered.
Hydromorphone opioid analgesic	No reports on first trimester use. May cause neonatal CNS depression or withdrawal.	No neonatal safety data. Proposed monitoring: CNS depression, withdrawal.
Hydroxy-chloroquine antimalarial, antirheumatic	No apparent malformation risk in repeated small studies. See page 108	No apparent neonatal risk based on small numbers. Proposed monitoring: CNS excitation, cinchonism. Advantages of breastfeeding should be considered.
Hydroxy-progesterone	No apparent malformation risk for oral contraceptive based on meta-analyses.	No neonatal safety data. Advantages of breastfeeding should be considered.
Hydroxyurea anticancer	Cancer drugs inhibit cell division and may induce birth defects in first trimester. See page 150	Breastfed infants should not be exposed to cancer drugs through breast milk.
Hydroxyzine antihistamine	No apparent malformation risk based on repeated studies. No apparent malformation risk for H_1 blockers based on a large number of studies. See page 101	No apparent neonatal risk. Proposed monitoring: CNS depression. Advantages of breastfeeding should be considered.

(Continued)

	Pregnancy risk-benefit	Breastfeeding
Ibuprofen nonsteroidal anti-inflammatory	No apparent malformation risk based on repeated studies. A possible increased risk for miscarriage. NSAIDs may cause premature closure of ductus arteriosus. See pages 154, 242	No apparent neonatal risk based on small numbers. Advantages of breastfeeding should be considered.
Ibulitide antiarrhythmic	No human data. There are antiarrhythmics with fetal safety data.	No human data. Proposed monitoring: heart rate.
Idarubicin anticancer	Cancer drugs inhibit cell division and may cause birth defects in first trimester. See page 150	Neonates should not be exposed to cancer drugs through breast milk. Advantages of breastfeeding should be considered.
Ifosfamide anticancer	Cancer drugs inhibit cell division and may cause birth defects in first trimester. See page 150	Neonates should not be exposed to cancer drugs through breast milk.
Imipenem antibiotic	No reports on first trimester exposure. No apparent malformation risk for penicillins based on large numbers.	Small amounts in milk. Proposed monitoring: diarrhea due to potential change in gut flora. Advantages of breastfeeding should be considered.
Imipramine antidepressant	No apparent malformation risk or developmental delay in repeated studies. The neonate may exhibit poor neonatal adaptation syndrome. Untreated depression increases perinatal risks. See pages 290, 293, 297	No apparent neonatal risk based on small numbers. Advantages of breastfeeding should be considered.

(Continued)

	Pregnancy risk-benefit	Breastfeeding
Indinavir anti-HIV	No apparent malformation risk based on small numbers. See page 312	HIV may infect the infant through breast milk.
Indomethacin nonsteroidal anti-inflammatory	No apparent malformation risk based on small numbers. When used at term—oligohydramnios and neonatal decrease in renal function may occur. May cause premature closure of ductus arteriosus. See pages 154, 242	Small amounts in milk. No data on neonatal safety. Given at large dose to neonates to close ductus arteriosus. Advantages of breastfeeding should be considered.
Infliximab antirheumatic	An antibody; unlikely to cross the placenta at appreciable amounts. No adequate safety data in first trimester.	No human data. The drug, even if enters milk, unlikely to be absorbed unchanged by the infant.
Insulin	Marginal placental transfer. No apparent malformation risk due to insulin. Untreated diabetes increases malformation risk.	Does not cross into milk.
Interferon, alfa immunologic	Probably does not cross the placenta. No apparent malformation risk based on small numbers.	No neonatal safety data. Advantages of breastfeeding should be considered.
Interferon, beta immunologic	No apparent malformation risk based on small numbers. May increase risk of miscarriages.	No human data. Advantages of breastfeeding should be considered.
Ipratropium anticholinergic antiasthmatic	Used by inhalation. No apparent malformation risk based on small numbers.	No human data. Advantages of breastfeeding should be considered.

(Continued)

	Pregnancy risk-benefit	Breastfeeding
Irbesartan antihypertensive	Angiotensin II receptor antagonists can cause fetal/neonatal renal insufficiency, oligohydramnion and hypocalciuria when used in second to third trimesters.	No human data.
Isoetharine sympathomimetic	No apparent malformation risk based on small numbers.	No human data. Proposed monitoring: heart rate, blood pressure.
Isoflurane inhaled anesthetic	No fetal safety data in first trimester. No apparent risk when used at term. Occupational exposure to inhaled anesthetics-increased miscarriage risk. See page 231	No human data. Proposed monitoring: CNS depression.
Isoniazid anti-TB	No apparent malformation risk based on small numbers. Maternal TB should be treated.	No neonatal safety data. Small amounts in milk. Advantages of breastfeeding should be considered.
Isoproterenol sympathomimetic	No apparent malformation risk based on small numbers.	No human data. Proposed monitoring: heart rate, blood pressure. Advantages of breastfeeding should be considered.
Isosorbide diuretic	No apparent malformation risk based on small numbers.	No human data. Proposed monitoring: urine output. Advantages of breastfeeding should be considered.

(Continued)

	Pregnancy risk-benefit	Breastfeeding
Isosorbide dinitrate vasodilator	No fetal safety data.	No human data. Advantages of breastfeeding should be considered.
Isotretinoin antiacne	Causes high rates of retinoid embryopathy: CNS, ear, eye, face, cardiovascular malformations. See pages 251, 256	No neonatal safety data.
Isoxsuprine vasodilator	No fetal data on first trimester. When used at term—no apparent fetal- neonatal risk based on relatively large numbers.	No human data. Proposed monitoring: heart rate, blood pressure. Advantages of breastfeeding should be considered.
Isradipine anti-hypertensive	No apparent malformation risk based on small numbers for this drug, or for calcium channel blockers in general.	No human data. Advantages of breastfeeding should be considered.
Itraconazole antifungal	No apparent malformation risk based on several studies.	No neonatal safety data. Advantages of breastfeeding should be considered.
Ivermectin antihelmintic	No apparent malformation risk in repeated studies.	No neonatal safety data. Advantages of breastfeeding should be considered.
Kanamycin aminogly-coside	No apparent malformation risk based on small numbers. Neonatal hearing loss has been rarely described in case reports, but no causation established.	Very small amounts in milk. Proposed monitoring: diarrhea, due to potential change in gut flora.

(Continued)

	Pregnancy risk-benefit	Breastfeeding
Ketamine anesthetic	No data on first trimester. Wide experience at term. May be oxytocic and may cause neonatal CNS depression.	No human data. Short half-life in mother (2 hours). Proposed monitoring: CNS depression.
Ketoconazole antifungal	No apparent malformation risk based on small numbers.	No human data. Advantages of breastfeeding should be considered.
Ketoprofen nonsteroidal anti-inflammatory	No apparent malformation risk in small numbers. NSAIDs may cause tocolysis and premature closure of the ductus arteriosus near term. See pages 154, 242	No human data. Advantages of breastfeeding should be considered.
Ketorolac Nonsteroidal anti-inflammatory	No safety data on first trimester use. NSAIDs may cause tocolysis and premature closure of the ductus arteriosus near term. See pages 154, 242	No neonatal safety data. Advantages of breastfeeding must be considered.
Labetalol antihypertensive	No apparent malformation risk based on small numbers. No developmental delays in a controlled study. No apparent neonatal risk when used at term.	No apparent neonatal risk based on small numbers. Advantages of breastfeeding should be considered.
Laetrile anticancer	No fetal safety data. Laetril leads to cyanide production. Cyanide is teratogenic. See page 150	No human data.

(Continued)

	Pregnancy risk-benefit	Breastfeeding
Lamivudine anti-HIV	No apparent malformation risk based on small numbers. Neonatal mitochondrial disease was described in some preliminary studies but was not corroborated. See page 312	Babies may contract HIV through breastfeeding.
Lamotrigine antiepileptic	No apparent malformation risk based on several studies.	No apparent neonatal risk based on small numbers. Advantages of breastfeeding should be considered.
Lansoprazole proton pump inhibitor	No apparent malformation risk in small numbers. Proton pumps as a group do not appear to increase malformation risk (based on meta-analysis).	No human data. Potential suppression of gastric acid secretion. Advantages of breastfeeding should be considered.
Leflunamide antirheumatic	Cause high rates of malformations in animals at blood levels similar to clinical concentration. No apparent risk in a small prospective human study.	No human data.
Lepirudin thrombin inhibitor	A large molecule that probably cannot cross the placenta or cross at low levels. No safety in first trimester.	No human data. Even if appears in milk—unlikely to be absorbed intact.
Leuprolide anticancer hormone	Suppresses endometrial proliferation. No apparent malformation risk based on small numbers.	No human data.

(Continued)

	Pregnancy risk-benefit	Breastfeeding
Levallorphan opioid antagonist	No first trimester human data.	No human data.
Levetiracetam antiepileptic	No human data. There are fetal safety data on many other anticonvulsants.	No human data. Advantages of breastfeeding should be considered.
Levadopa antiparkin-sonism	No apparent malformation risk in small numbers.	No apparent neonatal risk based on small numbers. Advantages of breastfeeding should be considered.
Levofloxacin quinolone	No human data. There are quinolones with fetal safety data (e.g., ciprofloxacin, ofloxacin).	No human data. Proposed monitoring: diarrhea due to change in gut flora. Advantages of breastfeeding should be considered.
Levothyroxine thyroid hormone	Safe in pregnancy. Low levels of thyroxine may adversely affect fetal brain development. See page 262	Safe.
Lidocaine local anesthetic, antiarrhythmic	No apparent malformation risk based on several studies.	Small amounts in milk. No data on neonatal safety. Advantages of breastfeeding should be considered. Proposed monitoring: heart rate.
Lincomycin antibiotic	No apparent malformation risk based on one relatively large study.	No apparent neonatal risk. Proposed monitoring: diarrhea due to potential change in gut flora.

(Continued)

	Pregnancy risk-benefit	Breastfeeding
Lindane scabicide	Used topically. No apparent malformation risk based on large data.	No data. Advantages of breastfeeding should be considered.
Linezolid antibacterial	No human data. There are scores of antibiotics with fetal safety data.	No human data. Proposed monitoring: diarrhea, due to potential change in gut flora.
Liothyroxin T$_3$	A normal constituent in blood. Safe in pregnancy. Low levels are associated with neurodevelopmental deficits. See page 262	Normal constituent. Safe.
Lipids parenteral nutrition	No apparent malformation risk based on small numbers.	No human data. Advantages of breastfeeding should be considered.
Lisinopril antihypertensive	angiotensin-converting enzyme (ACE) inhibitors, including lisinopril can cause fetal renal insufficiency, oligohydramnion and hypocalvaria in third trimester. No apparent malformation risk in first trimester based on small numbers. See pages 198, 204	No human data. Advantages of breastfeeding should be considered. Proposed monitoring: blood pressure, urinary output, renal function.
Lithium for manic depression	Can cause Epstein anomaly (tricuspid insufficiency) in less than 1% of babies. At term, some babies may experience transient cyanosis, hypotonia, hypothyroidism, bradycardia.	May accumulate in large amounts in some cases but not other. Proposed monitoring: measure lithium in milk and in baby's blood if adverse effects are suspected.

(Continued)

	Pregnancy risk-benefit	Breastfeeding
Lomefloxacin quinolone	No human data. No apparent malformation risk for quinolones as a group based on several studies.	No human data. Proposed monitoring: diarrhea due to potential change in gut flora.
Loperamide antidiarrheal	No apparent malformation risk based on small numbers.	No human studies. Advantages of breastfeeding should be considered.
Lopinovir anti-HIV	No apparent malformation risk based on small numbers. See page 312	HIV may transfer to baby through milk.
Loracarbef antibiotic beta-lactam	No human data. No apparent malformation risk for penicillin based on large numbers.	No human data. Proposed monitoring: diarrhea due to potential change in gut flora.
Loratadine antihistamine	No apparent malformation risk based on several studies. No apparent malformation risk for antihistamines in general based on large studies. See page 161	No apparent neonatal risk based on small numbers. Advantages of breastfeeding should be considered.
Lorazepam benzodiazepine	No apparent malformation risk based on small numbers. No apparent malformation risk for benzodiazepines, except for unclear risk of oral cleft. Neonatal withdrawal may occur at term. See page 184	May cause sedation. Proposed monitoring: CNS depression.

(Continued)

	Pregnancy risk-benefit	Breastfeeding
Losartan antihyper-tensive	Angiotensin II antagonist, similar to ACE inhibitors, may cause fetal renal insufficiency, oligohydramnion, and hypocalvaria. See page 159	No human data. Advantages of breastfeeding should be considered. Proposed monitoring: blood pressure.
Lovastatin antilipemic	Statins may disrupt fetal cholesterol metabolism. No apparent malformation risk based on small numbers. See page 159	No human data.
Loxapine tranquilizer	No human data. There are tranquilizers with fetal safety data.	No human data. Proposed monitoring: CNS depression.
Lysergic acid diethylamide (LSD)	No apparent malformation risk based on several studies. No knowledge on neurobehavioral development.	No human data. Proposed monitoring: CNS status.
Magnesium sulfate anticonvulsant	No apparent malformation risk based on small numbers. Used extensively at term with no apparent fetal risk.	No apparent neonatal risk based on small numbers. Advantages of breastfeeding should be considered.
Mandelic acid urinary antibacterial	No apparent malformation risk based on small numbers.	No report on neonatal safety. Proposed monitoring: diarrhea due to potential change in gut flora. Advantages of breastfeeding should be considered.

(*Continued*)

	Pregnancy risk-benefit	Breastfeeding
Maprotiline antidepressant	No apparent malformation risk based on small numbers. There are antidepressants with much larger fetal safety data. See pages 290, 293, 297	No report on neonatal safety. Advantages of breastfeeding should be considered.
Marijuana psychoactive drug of abuse	No apparent malformation risk based on many studies. Possible adverse effects on neurodevelopment. See page 266	No apparent neonatal risk based on small numbers. May affect neonatal CNS. See page 271
Mebendazole anthelmintic	No apparent malformation risk based on small numbers.	Small amounts in milk. No neonatal safety data.
Mechlorethane anticancer	Cancer drugs inhibit cell proliferation and may affect the embryo during first trimester. See page 150	Infants should not be exposed to cancer drugs through milk.
Meclizine antihistamine-antiemetic	No apparent malformation risk based on large numbers.	No human data. Advantages of breastfeeding should be considered.
Meclofenamate nonsteroidal anti-inflammatory	No apparent malformation risk in small numbers. NSAIDs may cause premature closure of the ductus arteriosus in late pregnancy. See pages 154, 242	No human data. Advantages of breastfeeding should be considered.
Medroxyproges-terone	No apparent teratogenic risk for progestins based on many studies and meta-analysis.	No risk for progestenic hormones during lactation.

(Continued)

	Pregnancy risk-benefit	Breastfeeding
Mefenamic acid nonsteroidal anti-inflammatory	No apparent malformation risk based on small numbers. NSAIDs may cause premature closure of the ductus arteriosus in late pregnancy. See pages 154, 242	Small amounts in milk. No apparent neonatal risk based on small numbers.
Mefloquine antimalarial	No apparent malformation risk based on several studies. See page 168	No studies on neonatal risk.
Melatonin	No published safety data with exogenous use.	No studies on neonatal risk.
Melphalan anticancer	Anticancer drugs inhibit cell proliferation, and hence may induce birth defects in first trimester. See page 150	Infants should not be exposed to cancer drugs through milk.
Meperidine opioid	No apparent malformation risk based on several studies. Neonatal withdrawal may occur at term.	No apparent neonatal risk reported. Proposed monitoring: CNS depression.
Mephobarbital antiepileptic, sedative	No apparent malformation risk based on small numbers. Neonatal withdrawal may occur.	No human data. Proposed monitoring: CNS depression.
Meprobamate sedative	No apparent malformation risk in several studies. Neonatal withdrawal may occur. See page 184	No reports of neonatal safety. Proposed monitoring: CNS depression.

(Continued)

	Pregnancy risk-benefit	Breastfeeding
Mercaptopurine anticancer	Anticancer drug inhibits cell proliferation and may produce congenital malformations in first trimester. No apparent malformation risk based on small numbers and experience with azathioprine.	No human data. The infant should not be exposed to cancer drugs through milk.
Mesalamine anti-inflammatory bowel disease	No apparent malformation risk based on several studies.	Description of diarrhea in a breastfed baby. Small amounts in breast milk. Proposed monitoring: gastrointestinal symptoms. Advantages of breastfeeding should be considered.
Mestranol estrogen	No apparent malformation risk to estrogens based on several meta-analyses.	May decrease milk production. Advantages of breastfeeding should be considered.
Metaproteronol sympath-omimetic	No apparent malformation risk based on small numbers. When used at term—no apparent fetal risk.	No human data. Advantages of breastfeeding should be considered.
Metaxalone muscle relaxant	No published safety data in first trimester.	No human data. Advantages of breastfeeding should be considered.
Metformin oral hypoglycemic	No apparent malformation risk based on meta-analysis. See page 274	Small amounts in milk. No neonatal safety data. Advantages of breastfeeding should be considered.

(Continued)

	Pregnancy risk-benefit	Breastfeeding
Methadone opioid	No apparent malformation risk in several studies. Neonatal withdrawal may occur.	No apparent neonatal risk. Small amounts in milk. Proposed monitoring: CNS depression, neonatal withdrawal.
Methaqualone hypnotic	No human data.	No human data. Proposed monitoring: CNS depression.
Methenamine urinary antibacterial	No apparent malformation risk based on small numbers.	No reports of neonatal safety. Proposed monitoring: diarrhea due to potential change in gut flora.
Methimazole antithyroid	May increase the risk for aplasia cutis. No apparent risk of neurobehavioral deficits. See page 202	No apparent neonatal risk. Advantages of breastfeeding should be considered.
Methocarbamol muscle relaxant	No apparent malformation risk based on several studies.	No human data. Advantages of breastfeeding should be considered.
Methotrexate anticancer	Can cause congenital malformations (fetal aminopterin-methotrexate syndrome): limb, CNS, oral cleft. See page 159	The infant should not be exposed to cancer drugs through milk.
Methoxsalen antipsoriasis (plus PUVA)	No apparent malformation rates based on small numbers.	No human data. Planned monitoring: psoralen ultraviolet A being a photosensitizer it may photosensitize the baby through milk.

(Continued)

	Pregnancy risk-benefit	Breastfeeding
Methyldopa antihypertensive	No apparent malformation risk based on several studies. At term, the neonate may exhibit beta-blockage.	No data on neonatal safety. Small amounts in milk. Advantages of breastfeeding should be considered.
Methylergonovine maleate oxytocic	No apparent malformation risk based on small numbers.	No neonatal safety data. Small amounts in milk (Hale). Advantages of breastfeeding should be considered.
Methylphenidate central stimulant	No apparent malformation risk based on small numbers. May cause neonatal withdrawal.	No neonatal safety data. Proposed monitoring: CNS stimulation.
Metoclopramide antiemetic	No apparent malformation risk based on several studies. See page 190	Can cause stimulation of lactation. No apparent neonatal risk. Proposed monitoring: gastrointestinal symptoms. Advantages of breastfeeding should be considered.
Metoprolol antihypertensive	No apparent malformation risk based on small numbers. Beta-blockers have been associated with intrauterine growth retardation. At term, the neonate may exhibit beta-blockage.	No neonatal safety data. Proposed monitoring: beta-blockade. Advantages of breastfeeding should be considered.
Metronidazole trichomonacide	No apparent malformation risk based on meta-analysis.	No apparent neonatal toxicity based on small numbers. Used in much larger doses in neonates. Advantages of breastfeeding should be considered.

(Continued)

	Pregnancy risk-benefit	Breastfeeding
Mexiletine antiarrhythmic	No apparent malformation based on small numbers.	No apparent toxicity based on small numbers. Advantages of breastfeeding should be considered.
Miconazole antifungal	No apparent malformation risk after vaginal use based on small numbers. Minimal systemic absorption.	No human data. Minimal systemic absorption. Advantages of breastfeeding should be considered.
Midazolam sedative	No first trimester data. At term—may cause neonatal CNS depression and poor adaptation. No apparent malformation risk for benzodiazepines, except for unclear risk of oral cleft. See page 184	No neonatal safety data. Proposed monitoring: CNS depression, poor adaptation. Advantages of breastfeeding should be considered.
Midodrine sympath- omimetic	No human data. There are sympathomimetics with fetal safety data (e.g., epinephrine, dopamine).	No human data. Advantages of breastfeeding should be considered.
Mifepristone abortifacient	Pregnant women should not be exposed to this potent antiprogestogen, except in the context of pregnancy termination.	No human data.
Miglitol oral hypoglycemic	No human data. There are oral hypoglycemics with fetal safety data (glyburide, metformin).	No neonatal safety data. Proposed monitoring: glucose levels.
Milrinone inotropic agent	No human data.	No human data.

(*Continued*)

	Pregnancy risk-benefit	Breastfeeding
Mineral oil laxative	Not absorbed in the gut. May decrease absorption of fat solubles vitamins D, E, K and A.	Safe, as it is not absorbed in the mother's gut.
Minocycline tetracycline	May cause discoloration and damage to teeth after $4\frac{1}{2}$ months gestation.	Small levels in milk. No apparent neonatal risks.
Minoxidil antihypertensive	No prospective data on first trimester. At term: neonatal hypotension and hypertrichosis with oral use.	No apparent neonatal risk based on few cases. Proposed monitoring: blood pressure.
Misoprostol gut antisecretory abortifacient	Causes the Moebius sequence (facial paralysis, limb anomalies, oral cleft) when used as abortifacient in first trimester.	No human data.
Mitoxantrone anticancer	Anticancer drugs inhibit cell development and may cause birth defects. See page 150	Breastfed infants should not be exposed to cancer drugs through milk.
Modafinil central stimulant	No human data.	No human data.
Moexipril antihypertensive	No apparent malformation risk based on small numbers. ACE inhibitors can cause fetal/neonatal renal insufficiency, oligohydramnios, and hypocalvaria in late pregnancy.	No human data. Proposed monitoring: blood pressure, urine output. Advantages of breastfeeding should be considered.
Montelukast antiasthma	No apparent malformation risk based on small numbers.	No human data. Advantages of breastfeeding should be considered.

(Continued)

	Pregnancy risk-benefit	Breastfeeding
Morphine opioid analgesic	No apparent malformation risk based on small numbers. At term—neonatal withdrawal may occur.	No apparent toxicity based on small numbers. Proposed monitoring: CNS depression.
Moxalactam cephalosporin	No human data during first trimester. No apparent malformation risk for cephalosporins as a group in several studies	No data on neonatal safety. Proposed monitoring: diarrhea due to potential change in gut flora.
Moxifloxacin quinolone	No human data. No apparent malformation risk for quinolones a group based on several studies.	No human data. Proposed monitoring: diarrhea due to potential change in gut flora.
Mycophenolate-mofetil immuno-suppressive	No prospective human data. There are antirejection drugs with fetal safety data (e.g., cyclosporine).	No human data. Advantages of breastfeeding should be considered.
Nabumetone Nonsteroidal anti-inflammatory	No human data. At term, NSAIDs may cause premature closure of the ductus arteriosus. See pages 154, 242	No human data. Advantages of breastfeeding should be considered.
Nadolol antihyper-tensive	No apparent malformation risk based on small numbers. Beta-blockers have been associated with intrauterine growth retardation. At term, the neonate may exhibit beta-blockage.	No neonatal safety data. Small amounts in milk. Proposed monitoring: blood pressure.
Nadroparin anticoagulant	Does not cross the human placenta. See page 208	Unlikely to appear in milk.

(Continued)

	Pregnancy risk-benefit	Breastfeeding
Nafcillin penicillin	No first trimester reports. No apparent malformation risk for penicillins as a group based on large numbers.	No human data. Proposed monitoring: diarrhea due to potential changes in gut flora. Advantages of breastfeeding should be considered.
Nalbuphine opioid agonist antagonist	No first trimester data. At term—may cause neonatal withdrawal.	No human data. Proposed monitoring: CNS depression.
Nalidixic acid urinary bacteriocide	No human data in first trimester.	No neonatal safety data. Proposed monitoring: diarrhea due to potential change in gut flora.
Nalorphine opioid antagonist	No data on first trimester use. No adverse fetal effects at term. No apparent risk for opioids as a group.	No human data.
Naloxone opioid antagonist	No data on first trimester use. No adverse fetal effects at term. No apparent risk for opioids as a group	No human data.
Naltrexone opioid antagonist	No data on first trimester exposure, or in late pregnancy. No apparent risk for opioids as a group	No human data.
Naproxen nonsteroidal anti-inflammatory	No apparent malformation risk based on large numbers. NSAIDs may cause premature closure of ductus arteriosus at term.	No apparent neonatal risk based on small numbers with short-term use. Advantages of breastfeeding should be considered.

(Continued)

	Pregnancy risk-benefit	Breastfeeding
Naratriptan antimigraine	No human data. There are drugs from this class with fetal safety data (e.g., sumatriptan)	No human data. Advantages of breastfeeding should be considered.
Nateglinide oral hypoglycemic	No human data. There are drugs from this class with fetal safety data (e.g., glyburide, metformin).	No human data. Advantages of breastfeeding should be considered. Proposed monitoring: blood glucose.
Nedocromil sodium anti-asthma	No apparent malformation risk based on small numbers. Minimal systemic absorption.	No human data. Minimal systemic absorption. Unlikely to appear in milk (Briggs). Advantages of breastfeeding should be considered.
Nefazodone antidepressant	No apparent malformation risk based on small numbers. Poor adaptation syndrome may occur at term.	No neonatal safety data. Advantages of breastfeeding should be considered.
Nelfinavir anti-HIV	No apparent malformation risk based on several studies. See page 312	HIV may be transmitted to the baby through breast milk.
Neomycin aminoglycoside	Minimal systemic absorption. No apparent malformation risk based on small numbers.	Unlikely to appear in milk. Proposed monitoring: diarrhea due to potential change in gut flora. Advantages of breastfeeding should be considered.
Neostigmine cholinergic	No apparent malformation risk based on small numbers.	No data on neonatal safety. Advantages of breastfeeding should be considered.

(Continued)

	Pregnancy risk-benefit	Breastfeeding
Nevirapine anti-HIV	No apparent malformation risk based on several studies. See page 312	HIV may be transmitted to the baby through breast milk.
Nicardipine calcium channel blocker (antianginal and hypertension)	No human data in first trimester. There are drugs from this class with fetal safety data (e.g., nifedipine).	No human data. Advantages of breastfeeding should be considered. Proposed monitoring: blood pressure.
Nicotine replacement antismoking	No evidence of teratogenicity in several studies See page 171	No human data. Advantages of breastfeeding should be considered.
Nifedipine calcium channel antihyper-tensive	No apparent malformation risk based on several studies.	No neonatal safety data. Advantages of breastfeeding should be considered. Small amounts in milk.
Nimodipine calcium channel blocker	No apparent malformation risk based on small numbers. There are drugs from this class with fetal safety data (e.g., nifedipine).	No neonatal safety data. Small amounts in milk. Advantages of breastfeeding should be considered. Proposed monitoring: blood pressure.
Nitazoxanide antiprotozoal	No human data.	No human data. Advantages of breastfeeding should be considered.
Nitrofurantoin antibacterial	No apparent malformation risk based on meta-analysis.	No apparent neonatal risk based on small numbers. Advantages of breastfeeding should be considered. Proposed monitoring: diarrhea due to potential change in gut flora.

(Continued)

	Pregnancy risk-benefit	Breastfeeding
Nitroglycerin vasodilator	No apparent malformation risk based on small numbers.	No human data. Advantages of breastfeeding should be considered. Proposed monitoring: blood pressure.
Nitroprusside antihypertensive	No first trimester experience.	No human data. Proposed monitoring: blood pressure.
Nitrous oxide anesthetic	No apparent malformation risk based on large number of studies. Chronic occupational exposure—risk of miscarriage—when good scavenging systems are absent.	No human data. Very short half-life in blood (3 minutes).
Nizatidine H_2 antagonist	No first trimester data. As a group—no apparent malformation risk with H_2 blockers based on several studies.	No neonatal safety data. Proposed monitoring: gastrointestinal symptoms.
Nonoxynol-9 spermicide	No apparent malformation risk based on meta-analysis. See page 278	No human data. Unlikely to appear in milk. Advantages of breastfeeding should be considered.
Norepinephrine sympathomimetic	No data on first trimester use.	No human data. Advantages of breastfeeding should be considered.
Norethindrone progestogenic hormone	No apparent malformation risk for based on meta-analyses.	No apparent neonatal risk based on small numbers. Advantages of breastfeeding should be considered.

(Continued)

	Pregnancy risk-benefit	Breastfeeding
Norethynodrel progestogenic hormone	No apparent malformation risk for progesterone based on meta-analyses.	No apparent neonatal risk based on small numbers. Advantages of breastfeeding should be considered.
Norfloxacin quinolone	No apparent malformation risk based on several studies.	No human data. Proposed monitoring: diarrhea, due to potential change in gut flora. Advantages of breastfeeding should be considered.
Nortriptyline antidepressant	No apparent malformation or neurobehavioral risks, based on several studies. When used at term, poor neonatal adaptation syndrome may occur. See pages 290, 293, 297	No apparent neonatal risk. Advantages of breastfeeding should be considered.
Novobiocin antibiotics	No apparent malformation risk based on small numbers. See page 194	No data on neonatal safety. Proposed monitoring: diarrhea, due to potential change in gut flora.
Nutmeg herb	No human data, except of overdose with normal outcome.	No human data. Advantages of breastfeeding should be considered.
Nystatin antifungal	No apparent malformation risk based on one large study.	Poor absorption. No human data. Unlikely to appear in milk. Advantages of breastfeeding should be considered.

(Continued)

	Pregnancy risk-benefit	Breastfeeding
Octreotide somatostatin analogue	No apparent teratogenic risk based on small numbers.	No human data. Advantages of breastfeeding should be considered.
Ofloxacin quinolone	No apparent malformation risk based on small numbers. No apparent malformation risk for quinolones as a group based on several studies.	No neonatal safety data. Proposed monitoring: diarrhea due to potential change in gut flora.
Olanzapine atypical antipsychotic	No apparent malformation risk based on several studies. Excessive maternal weight gain and its complications may occur.	No apparent neonatal risk based on small numbers. Proposed monitoring: CNS depression. Advantages of breastfeeding should be considered.
Olmesartan antihyper-tensive	Angiotensin II antagonist can cause fetal renal insufficiency, oligohydramnion, and hypocalvaria in late pregnancy.	No human data. Proposed monitoring: blood pressure.
Omeprazole antisecretory	No apparent malformation risk based on several studies. No apparent malformation risk for proton pump inhibitors as a class based on meta-analysis. See page 281	No apparent neonatal risk based on a few cases. Advantages of breastfeeding should be considered.
Ondansetron antiemetic	No apparent malformation risk based on several studies. See page 281	No human data. Advantages of breastfeeding should be considered.
Oprelvekin hematopoietic	No human data.	No human data.

(Continued)

	Pregnancy risk-benefit	Breastfeeding
Oral contraceptives estrogen/ progestogenic combination	No apparent malformation risk based on meta-analysis.	No apparent neonatal risk. Advantages of breastfeeding should be considered.
Orlistat lipase inhibitor	No human data. See page 159	No human data. Advantages of breastfeeding should be considered.
Orphenadrine muscle relaxant	No apparent malformation risk based on one large study.	No human data. Advantages of breastfeeding should be considered.
Oxacillin penicillin	No apparent malformation risk based on several studies. No apparent malformation risk for penicillins based on large numbers.	No apparent neonatal risk. Proposed monitoring: diarrhea due to potential change in gut flora.
Oxazepam sedative	No apparent malformation risk for benzodiazepines based on meta-analysis, except for unclear association with oral cleft. When used at term neonatal sedation or withdrawal can occur. See page 184	No neonatal safety data. Proposed monitoring: CNS depression.
Oxcarbazepine antiepileptic	No apparent teratogenic risk based on small numbers.	No apparent neonatal risk based on a case report. Advantages of breastfeeding should be considered.

(Continued)

	Pregnancy risk-benefit	Breastfeeding
Oxprenolol antihypertensive	No data on first trimester. There are beta-blockers with fetal safety data (e.g., labetalol, atenolol, propranolol).	No neonatal safety data. Proposed monitoring: blood pressure and heart rate. Advantages of breastfeeding should be considered.
Oxybutynin urinary antispasmodic	No human data.	No human data. Advantages of breastfeeding should be considered.
Oxycodone opioid analgesic	No apparent malformation risk based on small numbers. Neonatal CNS depression or withdrawal can occur when used at term.	No neonatal safety data. Proposed monitoring: CNS depression.
Oxmetazoline symphthomimetic nasal decongestant	No apparent malformation risk based on small numbers. Minimal systemic absorption.	No human data. Milk levels after maternal nasal spray—probably negligible. Advantages of breastfeeding should be considered.
Paclitaxel anticancer	Cancer drugs inhibit cell development and proliferation, and can cause cong. malformation when used in first trimester. See page 150	Breastfed neonates should not be exposed to cancer drugs through maternal milk.
Pancuronium neuromuscular blocker	No reports on first trimester. Used safety in fetal injections for various procedures.	No human data. Advantages of breastfeeding should be considered.

(*Continued*)

	Pregnancy risk-benefit	Breastfeeding
Paramethadione antiepileptic	Causes malformations in first trimester (trimethadione syndrome): growth retardation, cardiac CNS, limb, urogenital.	No human data.
Parnaparin anticoagulant	Does not cross the placenta. See page 208	No neonatal safety data. Probably does not appear in milk.
Paroxetine antidepressant	No apparent malformation risk or neurocognitive effects based on several studies and meta-analysis. At term: poor neonatal adaptation syndrome may occur. See pages 286, 290, 293	No apparent neonatal risk based on small numbers. Proposed monitoring: poor adaptation syndrome. Advantages of breastfeeding should be considered.
Passion flower herb	No human data. See page 194	No human data. Advantages of breastfeeding should be considered.
Penicillamine chelator	Associated with cutis laxa in several cases.	No human data.
Penicillin antibiotic	No apparent malformation risk based on large numbers.	No apparent neonatal risk. Advantages of breastfeeding should be considered.
Pentamidine antiprotozoal	No reports on first trimester use.	If used in HIV patients— breastfeeding is contraindicated due to HIV passage to milk.

(Continued)

	Pregnancy risk-benefit	Breastfeeding
Pentazocine opioid agonist-antagonist	No apparent malformation risk based on several studies. Infants may exhibit withdrawal syndrome.	No human data. Proposed monitoring: CNS depression or withdrawal.
Pentobarbital sedative hypnotic	No apparent malformation risk based on several studies. When used at term—neonatal withdrawal or CNS depression may occur.	No neonatal safety data. Proposed monitoring: CNS depression.
Pentoxifylline hematologic	No apparent malformation risk based on small numbers.	No neonatal safety data. Advantages of breastfeeding should be considered.
Pergolide antiparkinsonian	No human data beyond one case report.	No human data.
Permethrin antiscabies	Topical drug likely not reaching the fetus.	Topical use likely not reaching the milk in relevant amounts. No apparent neonatal risk.
Perphenazine tranquilizer	No apparent malformation risk based on small numbers. No apparent malformation risk for phenothiazines based on meta-analysis.	No apparent neonatal toxicity based on small numbers. Proposed monitoring: CNS depression.
Phenacetin analgesic	No apparent malformation risk based on large numbers.	No neonatal safety data. Advantages of breastfeeding should be considered.
Phencyclidine hallucinogen	No apparent malformation risk based on small numbers. At term—poor neonatal adaptation may occur.	No neonatal safety data.

(Continued)

	Pregnancy risk-benefit	Breastfeeding
Phenelzine antidepressants	Very limited human data with no clear effect on monoamine oxidase (MAO) inhibitors. There are newer classes of antidepressants with large fetal safety data (SSRIs, selective norepinephrine reuptake inhibitor [SNRIs], tricyclics). See pages 290, 293, 297	No human data.
Pheniramine antihistamine	One large study suggested association with eye/ear defects. Not confirmed by meta-analyses. See page 161	No human studies. Proposed monitoring: CNS depression.
Phenobarbital sedative/ antiepileptic	An apparent neurocognitive effect on cohorts and randomized trials. When used at term—neonatal withdrawal or CNS depression may occur.	Phenobarbital is excreted in large amounts into milk. Proposed monitoring: CNS depression.
Phenoxy-benzamine antihyper-tensive	No reports on first trimester use.	No human data.
Phentermine anorexiant	No data on first trimester use.	No human reports.
Phentolamine antihyper-tensive	No apparent risk based on a few cases.	No human data.
Phenylbutazone nonsteroidal anti-inflammatory	No apparent malformation risk based on small numbers. NSAIDs can cause premature closure of the ductus arteriosus. See pages 154, 242	No apparent neonatal risks based on a case report. Advantages of breastfeeding should be considered.

(Continued)

	Pregnancy risk-benefit	Breastfeeding
Phenylephrine sympathomimetic	No apparent malformation risk based on a large study. Association was suggested with minor anomalies.	No human data. Advantages of breastfeeding should be considered.
Phenylpropanolamine sympathomimetic	No apparent malformation risk based on a large study. Association was suggested with minor anomalies. Case control studies suggested association with gastroschisis.	No human data. Advantages of breastfeeding should be considered.
Phenytoin antiepileptic	Causes the fetal hydantoin syndrome: decreased IQ, facial changes, small-absent nails, hypoplastic distal phalanges.	No apparent neonatal risk in small numbers. Advantages of breastfeeding should be considered.
Phytonadione vitamin K_1	No apparent malformation risk based on small numbers.	Safe.
Pimozide antipsychotic	No human data. There are antipsychotics with fetal safety data (both typical and atypical antipsychotics).	No human data. Proposed monitoring: CNS depression.
Pindolol antihypertensive	No data on first trimester exposure. When exposed later—beta-blockers were associated with intrauterine growth retardation.	No human data. Proposed monitoring: blood pressure, heart rate. Advantages of breastfeeding should be considered.
Proglitozone oral hypoglycemic	No human data. There are hypoglycemics with fetal safety data (e.g., glyburide, metformin).	No human data. Proposed monitoring: blood glucose. Advantages of breastfeeding should be considered.

(*Continued*)

	Pregnancy risk-benefit	Breastfeeding
Piperacillin (penicillin)	No first trimester exposure. No apparent malformation risk for penicillins based on large numbers.	No human reports. Proposed monitoring: diarrhea due to potential change in gut flora. Advantages of breastfeeding should be considered.
Piperazine anthelmintic	No apparent malformation risk based on small numbers.	No neonatal safety data. Advantages of breastfeeding should be considered.
Piroxicam nonsteroidal anti-inflammatory	No apparent malformation risk based on small numbers. NSAIDs may cause premature closure of the ductus arteriosus. See pages 154, 242	No neonatal safety data. Advantages of breastfeeding should be considered.
Podophyllum keratolytic	Few malformations in case reports. No controlled data.	No human data.
Potassium iodide expectorant	Iodine may cause fetal hypothyroidism and goiter. Ensure you know when you give iodine-containing drugs to pregnant women.	Iodine concentrate in milk. Proposed monitoring: thyroid function.
Promipexole antiparkin-sonian	No human data.	No human data. Proposed monitoring: CNS status.
Pravastatin antilipemic	Statins may affect fetal development by interruption of cholesterol metabolism.	No human data.
Praziquantel anthelmintic	No human data.	No human data.

(Continued)

	Pregnancy risk-benefit	Breastfeeding
Prazocin antihypertensive	No first trimester data. There are antihypertensives with fetal safety data (labetalol, methyldopa, atenolol, nifedipine).	No human data. Advantages of breastfeeding should be considered.
Prednisone/ prednisolone corticosteroid	May increase the risk of oral cleft in first trimester. See pages 154, 236	No apparent neonatal risk based on small numbers. Advantages of breastfeeding should be considered.
Primidone antiepileptics	Metabolized to phenobarbital, and hence has potential phenobarbital risks (see above).	No neonatal safety data. Proposed monitoring: CNS depression. Advantages of breastfeeding should be considered.
Probenecid inhibitor of organic acid secretion	No apparent malformation risk based on a large study.	No human data. Advantages of breastfeeding should be considered.
Procainamide antiarrhythmic	No apparent malformation risk based on case reports. Has been used safely for fetal dysrhythmias	No neonatal safety data. Proposed monitoring: heart rate.
Procarbazine anticancer	Anticancer drugs inhibit cell division and proliferation and may cause congenital defects. See pages 154, 236	Breastfed infants should not be exposed to cancer drugs through breast milk.
Prochlorperazine tranquilizer, antiemetic	No apparent malformation risk based on large numbers. At term—may cause CNS depression. See page 190	No human data. Proposed monitoring: CNS depression. Advantages of breastfeeding should be considered.

(Continued)

	Pregnancy risk-benefit	Breastfeeding
Proguanil antimalarial	No apparent malformation risk based on large numbers. See page 150	No neonatal safety data. Advantages of breastfeeding should be considered.
Promazine tranquilizer	No apparent malformation risk based on small numbers. No apparent malformation risk for phenothiazines based on meta-analysis.	No human data. Proposed monitoring: CNS depression. Advantages of breastfeeding should be considered.
Promethazine antihistamine	No apparent malformation risk based on large numbers. No apparent malformation risk for antihistamines as a group based on meta-analysis. See page 161	No human data. Proposed monitoring: CNS depression. Advantages of breastfeeding should be considered.
Propafenone antiarrhythmic	No first trimester experience.	No human data. Proposed monitoring: heart rate. Advantages of breastfeeding should be considered.
Propofol hypnotic	No first trimester data. At term—may cause neonatal CNS depression.	No neonatal safety data. Proposed monitoring: CNS depression.
Propoxyphene opioid agonist-antagonist	No apparent malformation rates based on large studies. When used at term—baby may have CNS depression or withdrawal.	No neonatal safety data. Proposed monitoring: CNS depression withdrawal.

(*Continued*)

	Pregnancy risk-benefit	Breastfeeding
Propranolol antihypertensive	No apparent malformation rate based on relatively large numbers. Beta-blockers are associated with intrauterine growth retardation, neonatal hypoglycemia, bradycardia.	No neonatal safety data. Proposed monitoring: heart rate, blood pressure, blood glucose. Advantages of breastfeeding should be considered.
Propylthiouracil antithyroid	No apparent malformation rate based on several small studies. Congenital thyroid goiter may develop. See page 262	No apparent neonatal risk based on several studies. Advantages of breastfeeding should be considered. Proposed monitoring: thyroid function.
Pseudoephedrine sympathomimetic	No apparent malformation risk based on large studies. Case control studies suggest association with gastroschisis.	No apparent neonatal risk based on small numbers. Advantages of breastfeeding should be considered.
Pyridostigmine cholinergic	No apparent malformation risk based on case reports.	No neonatal safety data. Minimal levels in milk. Proposed monitoring: muscular weakness.
Pyrimethamine antimalarial	No apparent malformation risk based on small numbers.	No neonatal safety data. Advantages of breastfeeding should be considered.
Quazepam hypnotic	No human data. No apparent malformation risk for benzodiazepines as a class, except for an unclear association with oral cleft. See page 184	No neonatal safety data. Proposed monitoring: CNS depression.

(Continued)

	Pregnancy risk-benefit	Breastfeeding
Quietapine atypical antipsychotic	No apparent malformation risk based on small numbers. Mother may experience weight gain and its complications.	No human data. Proposed monitoring: CNS depression. Advantages of breastfeeding should be considered.
Quinidine antiarrhythmic	No apparent malformation risk based on case reports.	No neonatal safety data. Proposed monitoring: heart rate. Advantages of breastfeeding should be considered.
Quinine antimalarial	No apparent malformation risk based on small numbers.	No apparent neonatal risk based on small numbers. Advantages of breastfeeding should be considered.
Rabeprazole GiT antisecretory	No first trimester data or late trimesters. There are proton pumpinhibitors with fetal safety data (e.g., omeprazole). See page 281	No human data.
Ramipril antihyper-tensive	No first trimester data or late trimesters. ACE inhibitors can cause fetal renal insufficiency, oligohydramion, and hypocalvaria.	No human data. Proposed monitoring: blood pressure, urine output.
Ranitidine antisecretory	No apparent malformation risk based on large numbers. See page 281	No neonatal safety data. Proposed monitoring: gastrointestinal symptoms. Advantages of breastfeeding should be considered.

(Continued)

	Pregnancy risk-benefit	Breastfeeding
Remifentanil opioid analgesic	No reports on first trimester exposure. At term may cause neonatal CNS depression or withdrawal.	No human data. Proposed monitoring: CNS depression withdrawal.
Repaglinide oral hypoglycemic	No human data in first or late trimesters. There are hypoglycemics with fetal safety data (e.g., glyburide, metformin).	No human data. Proposed monitoring: blood glucose.
Reviparin anticoagulant	Low molecular weight heparins do not cross the placenta. No apparent malformation risk in small numbers.	Unlikely to cross to milk. No neonatal safety data.
Ribarvirin antiviral	No first trimester experience in controlled studies.	No human data. Advantages of breastfeeding should be considered.
Rifampin anti-TB	No apparent malformation risk based on small numbers. Prophylaxis with vitamin K is recommended.	No neonatal safety data. Proposed monitoring: diarrhea due to potential change in gut flora. Advantages of breastfeeding should be considered.
Risperidone atypical antipsychotic	No apparent malformation risk based on small numbers. The woman may have excessive weight gain and its attendant risks.	Low milk levels based on small numbers. Proposed monitoring: CNS depression. Advantages of breastfeeding should be considered.

(*Continued*)

	Pregnancy risk-benefit	Breastfeeding
Ritodrin tocolytic	No first trimester exposure. Wide use for tocolysis with generally no apparent fetal/ neonatal risk.	No human data. Advantages of breastfeeding should be considered.
Ritonavir anti-HIV	No apparent malformation risk based on small numbers. See page 312	HIV may transfer to baby through breast milk.
Rizatriptan antimigraine	No apparent malformation risk based on small numbers. There are much larger numbers for sumatriptan, of the same class.	No human data. Advantages of breastfeeding should be considered.
Rocuronium neuroblocking	No first trimester data.	No human data. Proposed monitoring: muscular weakness.
Ropivacaine local anesthetic	No apparent malformation risk from local use.	No human data. Unlikely to reach milk when used locally as recommended.
Rosiglitazone oral hypoglycemic	No controlled reports on first trimester use. There are fetal safety data on other hypoglycemics (metformin glyburide).	No human data. Proposed monitoring: blood sugar.
Saccharin sweetener	No apparent malformation risk based on small numbers.	No apparent neonatal risk. Advantages of breastfeeding should be considered.

(Continued)

	Pregnancy risk-benefit	Breastfeeding
Salmeterol bronchodilator	No apparent malformation risk based on small numbers.	No human data. Unlikely that aerosolized drug enters milk in relevant amounts. Proposed monitoring: heart rate. Advantages of breastfeeding should be considered.
Saquinavir anti-HIV	No apparent malformation risk based on small numbers. See page 312	HIV may transfer to baby through breast milk.
Sargramostin hematspoietic	No human data.	No human data.
Scopolamine anticholinergic	No apparent malformation risk based on several studies.	No neonatal safety data. Proposed monitoring: heart rate. Advantages of breastfeeding should be considered.
Secobarbital	No apparent malformation risk based on a large study.	No neonatal safety data Proposed monitoring: heart rate.
Selegiline	No apparent risk based on case reports.	No human data. Animal data suggests neurotoxicity.
Senna herb laxative	No human data. See page 194	Diarrhea described in some babies. Proposed monitoring: diarrhea.
Sertraline antidepressant	No apparent malformation risk based on several studies and meta-analysis. A neonatal poor adaptation syndrome may occur. See pages 290, 293, 297	No apparent neonatal risk in small numbers. Proposed monitoring: CNS changes. Advantages of breastfeeding should be considered.

(Continued)

	Pregnancy risk-benefit	Breastfeeding
Sevelamer	No human data.	No human data.
Sevoflurane anesthetic	No first trimester reports. Occupational exposure associated with risk of miscarriage. Case report: no adverse effects when taken at 13 weeks (Reprotox). See page 231	No human data. Proposed monitoring: CNS depression.
Silicone breast implants	No apparent malformation risk or other anomalies based on small numbers.	No apparent neonatal risk based on small numbers.
Sibutramine	No human data. Weight loss in pregnancy not recommended.	No human data.
Simethicone antiflatulant	Not absorbed from the gut and therefore fetal-safe.	Unlikely to appear in milk.
Simvastatin	Statins inhibit cholesterol production and hence may affect fetal development. Small prospective studies do not show apparent malformation risk. See page 159	No human data. Other statins pass to milk (Briggs).
Sodium I^{131} radiophar-maceutical	May adversely affect fetal thyroid development.	May adversely affect thyroid development. Proposed monitoring: thyroid function.
Somatostatin	No risk based on small study (Reprotox).	No human data.
Sotalol antiarrhythmic	No first trimester data. Used in fetal arrhythmias. Beta-blockers are associated with intrauterine growth retardation.	No neonatal safety data. Proposed monitoring: beta-blockade. Advantages of breastfeeding should be considered.

(Continued)

	Pregnancy risk-benefit	Breastfeeding
Sparfloxacin quinolone	No human reports. No apparent teratogenic risk for quinolones as a group based on several studies.	No human data. Proposed monitoring: diarrhea due to potential change in gut flora. Advantages of breastfeeding should be considered.
Spectromycin	No human data.	No human data.
Spiramycin	No human data.	Limited human data. Likely compatible.
Spironolactone diuretics	No apparent malformation risk based on small numbers.	No neonatal safety data. Proposed monitoring: urine output. Advantages of breastfeeding should be considered.
Stavudine anti-HIV	No apparent malformation risk based on large numbers. See page 312	HIV may be transferred to the infant through milk.
St. John's wort herb— antidepressant	No apparent malformation risk based on small numbers. May affect metabolism of other drugs metabolized by CYP3A4. See page 301	No apparent neonatal risks based on small numbers. Advantages of breastfeeding should be considered.
Streptokinase thrombolytic	No apparent malformation risk based on small numbers.	No human data.
Streptomycin antibiotic	No apparent malformation risk based on small numbers.	No neonatal safety data. Proposed monitoring: diarrhea due to change in gut flora.

(Continued)

	Pregnancy risk-benefit	Breastfeeding
Succimer chelator	No human data.	No human data.
Succinylcholine muscle blockade agent	No data on first trimester. At term-may cause reversible neonatal paresis/paralysis.	No human data. Advantages of breastfeeding should be considered.
Sucralfate antisecretory	Very poor intestinal absorption. No apparent malformation risk based on small numbers. See page 281	No human data. Unlikely to reach milk. Advantages of breastfeeding should be considered.
Sufentanil opioid analgesic	No first trimester data. At term may cause neonatal CNS depression or withdrawal.	No human data. Proposed monitoring: CNS depression.
Sulbactam antibiotic	No first trimester data. No ↑ risk based on small numbers (second and third trimester) (Reprotox).	No neonatal safety data. Proposed monitoring: diarrhea due to change in gut flora. Advantages of breastfeeding should be considered.
Sulfasalazine for inflammatory bowel syndrome	No apparent malformation risk in several studies. As a folate antagonist— case control study associate increased risk for neural tube defects.	No neonatal safety data except for a case report with bloody diarrhea. Proposed monitoring: bowel movement. Advantages of breastfeeding should be considered.

(Continued)

	Pregnancy risk-benefit	Breastfeeding
Sulfonamides antibacterial	No apparent malformation risk in several cohort studies. Case control studies associate sulfonamides (antifolate agents) with neural tube defect. Theoretical concerns in third trimester use → kernicterus. See page 305	No apparent neonatal risk based on small numbers.
Sulindac nonsteroidal anti-inflammatory	No first trimester data. At term may cause premature closure of ductus arteriosus. See pages 154, 242	No reports. Advantages of breastfeeding should be considered.
Sumatriptan antimigraine	No apparent malformation risk based on several studies. The most extensively studied 5HT agonist.	No neonatal safety data. Advantages of breastfeeding should be considered.
Tacrolimus immuno-suppressant	No apparent malformation risk based on small numbers.	No apparent neonatal toxicity based on small numbers. Proposed monitoring: immunosuppression.
Tazarotene dermatologic agent	No apparent malformation risk based on small numbers. Systemic retinoids can cause malformations (CNS, ears, face, heart).	No neonatal safety studies.
Telmisartan antihyper-tensives	Angiotensin receptor antagonists can cause fetal renal insufficiency, oligohydramion, and hypocalvaria in late pregnancy. See pages 198, 204	No human data.

(Continued)

	Pregnancy risk-benefit	Breastfeeding
Temazepam hypnotic	No apparent malformation risk based on small numbers. At term— may cause CNS depression. For benzodiazepine—no apparent malformation risk based on meta-analysis, except for unclear association with oral cleft. See page 184	No neonatal safety data. Proposed monitoring: CNS depression.
Tenofovir anti-HIV	No apparent malformation risk based on small numbers. See page 312	HIV may be transferred to infant through milk.
Terbinafine antifungal	No human data.	No neonatal safety data.
Terbutaline antiasthmatic tocolytic	No apparent malformation risk based on small numbers. When used for tocolysis at term— may cause fetal tachycardia.	Inhalation is unlikely to yield high milk levels. Proposed monitoring: heart rate, blood pressure. Advantages of breastfeeding should be considered.
Terfenadine antihistamine	No apparent malformation risk based on large numbers. No apparent malformation risk for antihistamines as a group based on large numbers. See page 161	No apparent neonatal risk. Advantages of breastfeeding should be considered.
Testosterone androgenic hormone	May cause sexual changes in female fetuses (e.g., pseudohe-maphroditism).	May suppress lactation.

(Continued)

	Pregnancy risk-benefit	Breastfeeding
Tetanus toxoid	No apparent malformation risk in a case-control study.	No human data. The protein unlikely to appear in milk. Advantages of breastfeeding should be considered.
Tetracyclin antibiotic	May cause discoloration and damage to teeth after week 8 of gestation. No apparent malformation risk based on large numbers.	No apparent neonatal risks. Advantages of breastfeeding should be considered.
Thalidomide immunomodulator	Causes limb shortening defects, eye, ear, face, cardiovascular, gastrointestinal, renal, and genitourinary malformations.	No human data.
Theophylline antiasthma	No apparent malformation risk based on small numbers.	No controlled neonatal safety data. Proposed monitoring: CNS stimulation. Advantages of breastfeeding should be considered.
Thiobendazole anthelmintic	No human data.	No human data.
Thioguanine anticancer	Anticancer drugs inhibit cell division and proliferation and may cause birth defects in first trimester. See page 150	Infants should not be exposed to cancer drugs through milk.
Tiagabine antiepileptic	No human data.	No human data.

(*Continued*)

	Pregnancy risk-benefit	Breastfeeding
Ticarcillin penicillin	No human data. No apparent malformation risk with penicillins as a group based on large studies.	No neonatal safety data. Proposed monitoring: diarrhea due to potential change in gut flora. Advantages of breastfeeding should be considered.
Ticlopidine antiplatelets	No controlled human experience.	No human milk.
Timolol antihyper-tensive	No controlled human experience in first trimester. Beta-blockers are associated with intrauterine growth retardation. At term—neonatal bradycardia, hypoglycemia.	No apparent neonatal risk in a few cases. Proposed monitoring: heart rate, blood pressure. Advantages of breastfeeding should be considered.
Tinzaparin anticoagulant	Low molecular weight heparins do not cross the placenta. See page 208	No human data. Advantages of breastfeeding should be considered.
Tobramycin aminoglycoside	No apparent malformation risk based on small numbers.	No neonatal safety data. Proposed monitoring: diarrhea due to potential change in gut flora.
Tolazamide oral hypoglycemic	No apparent malformation risk based on meta-analysis. At term—neonatal hypoglycemia has been described.	No human data. Proposed monitoring: blood glucose.
Tolbutamide oral hypoglycemic	No apparent malformation risk based on meta-analysis. At term—neonatal hypoglycemia has been described.	No neonatal safety data. Proposed monitoring: blood glucose.

(Continued)

	Pregnancy risk-benefit	Breastfeeding
Tolmetin nonsteroidal anti-inflammatory	No apparent malformation risk based on small numbers. NSAIDs can cause premature closure of the ductus arteriosus at term. See pages 154, 242	No neonatal safety data. Advantages of breastfeeding should be considered.
Tolterodine urinary antisporradic	No human data.	No human data.
Topiramate antiepileptic	Uncontrolled, limited human data.	No apparent neonatal toxicity based on small numbers. Advantages of breastfeeding should be considered.
Trazodone antidepressant	No apparent malformation risk in several studies. At term may cause neonatal poor adaptation syndrome. See pages 290, 293, 297	No neonatal safety data. Advantages of breastfeeding should be considered.
Tretinoin (systemic) anticancer	May cause malformations similar to other retinoids (see isotretinoin).	No human data.
Tretinoin (topical) dermatologic	No apparent malformation risk based on several studies. See page 245	No human data.
Triamcinolone corticosteroid	No apparent malformation risk in small numbers. Case control studies show association between systemic corticosteroid and risk of oral cleft. See pages 154, 236	No human data.

(Continued)

	Pregnancy risk-benefit	Breastfeeding
Triamterene diuretic	No apparent malformation risk in one large study. Case control study suggest risk for neural tube and cardiac and oral cleft due to antifolic effect.	No human data. Proposed monitoring: urine output.
Triazolam hypnotic	No apparent malformation rate in several studies. Benzodiazepines are not associated with increased risk of malformation in meta-analysis, although for oral cleft association cannot be ruled out. At term—neonatal CNS depression or withdrawal. See page 184	No human data. Proposed monitoring: CNS depression.
Trifluoperazine tranquilizer	No apparent malformation risk in small numbers. No apparent malformation risk for phenothiazines in meta-analysis. At term—neonatal CNS	No human data. Proposed monitoring: CNS depression.
Trimethadione antiepileptic	May cause malformations (trimethadione syndrome), growth deficiency, mental retardation, facial defects, limb malformation, uregenital defects.	No human data.

(*Continued*)

	Pregnancy risk-benefit	Breastfeeding
Trimethoprim antibacterial	No clear malformation risk based on large numbers. Case control study suggests association with neural tube defects, oral clefts, and cardiac malformation due to antifolate effect.	No apparent neonatal risk. Proposed monitoring: diarrhea due to potential change in gut flora.
Tripelennamine antihistamine	No apparent malformation risk based on small numbers. No apparent malformation risk for antihistamines as a group based on large numbers. See page 161	No neonatal safety data. Proposed monitoring: sedation. Advantages of breastfeeding should be considered.
Troglitazone oral hypoglycemic	No first trimester experience.	No human data. Proposed monitoring: blood glucose.
Trovafloxacin quinolone	No human data. There are quinolones with fetal safety data (e.g., ciprofloxacin).	No neonatal safety data. Proposed monitoring: diarrhea due to change in gut flora. Advantages of breastfeeding should be considered.
Urokinase thrombolytic	No controlled human data. Case reports do not suggest malformation risk.	No human data. Very short half-life in mother (20 minutes or less).
Vaccines	<u>Anthrax</u>: Cell-free noninfectious. No plausible mechanism for fetal effects. No apparent malformation risk in large study. <u>BCG</u>: Live bacteria. No safety data. <u>Cholera</u>: No safety data.	No apperent neonatal risk. No human data. Increase in cholera IgA antibodies in milk.

(Continued)

	Pregnancy risk-benefit	Breastfeeding
	<u>E. Coli</u>: Non pathogenic strain. No adverse effects at term based on small numbers.	No apparent neonatal risk.
	<u>Group B Streptococcus</u>: Noninfectious. No adverse fetal effects in third trimester.	No human data.
	<u>Haemophilus B</u>: Noninfectious. No adverse fetal effects in third trimester.	Higher antibody titers in milk.
	<u>Hepatitis A</u>: Inactivated noninfectious vaccine. No safety data. Unlikely to affect the fetus.	No human data. Unlikely to be a problem for the newborn.
	<u>Hepatitis B</u>: Inactivated noninfectious antigens. No apparent fetal risk. No reports of fetal development anomalies.	No data. Unlikely to pose a problem to the neonate.
	<u>Influenza</u>: Inactive virus. No apparent fetal risk.	No apparent neonatal risk. Not contraindicated.
	See page 308 <u>Lyme Disease</u>: Noninfectious. No human reports. CDC collected 19 reported cases in pregnancy; in 14 instances→ no complications of pregnancy, five pregnancies complicated by prematurity, cardiac abnormalities, cortical blindness, fetal death.	No human data. Unlikely to pose a problem to the neonate. Shown that milk contained DNA from infective organism → no symptoms caused in infant
	<u>Measles</u>: Live vaccine. Fetal infection from the vaccine may occur.	No human data.
	<u>Meningococcus</u>: Killed bacteria. No apparent fetal risk based on small numbers.	No human data. Unlikely to pose a problem to the neonate.

(Continued)

	Pregnancy risk-benefit	Breastfeeding
	Mumps: Live attenuated virus. Fetal infection may occur. Recommend avoid becoming pregnant for 30 days postvaccine by CDC.	No human data. Unlikely to pose a problem to the neonate.
	Plague: Killed bacteria. No human data. Unlikely to pose fetal risk	No human data. Unlikely to pose a problem to the neonate.
	Pneumococcus: Killed bacteria. No apparent fetal risk in third trimester. Unborn risk in T1.	No human data. Unlikely to pose a problem to the neonate.
	Poliovirus: Inactivated. No apparent fetal risk.	No human data. Unlikely to pose a problem to the neonate.
	Oral Poliovirus: Live. No apparent fetal risk based large numbers.	No apparent neonatal risk.
	Rabies: Killed inactivated virus. No apparent fetal risk in small numbers.	No human data. Unlikely to pose a problem to the neonate.
	Rubella: Live attenuated virus. No apparent fetal risk based on several studies. No baby exhibited rubella syndrome.	No apparent neonatal risk.
	Smallpox: Live attenuated virus. May cause fetal infection.	No data. The attenuated virus may appear in milk.
	TC-83 Equine encephalitis: Live attenuated virus. May infect the fetus.	No human data.
	Tularemia: Live attenuated bacteria. Apparent safety in a single first trimester exposure.	No human data. Unlikely to pose a problem to the neonate.

(Continued)

	Pregnancy risk-benefit	Breastfeeding
	<u>Varicella</u>: Live attenuated virus. No apparent fetal risk based on small numbers.	No viral growth in milk.
	<u>Yellow Fever</u>: Live attenuated virus. No apparent fetal risk based on small numbers. Deter vaccination until T2 or T3.	No human data.
Valacyclovir antiviral	No apparent malformation risk based on small numbers. Not recommended as first line because of paucity of information.	No neonatal safety data.
Valdecoxib nonsteroidal anti- inflammatory	No human data. NSAIDs may cause premature closure of the ductus arteriosus.	No human data. Advantages of breastfeeding should be considered.
Valerian herb	No apparent malformation risk based on a few case reports.	No human data.
Valproic acid antiepileptic	Increase the risk of neural tube defects, cardiac anomalies, and limb malformation, and neurocognitive delays and liver damage but is rare. Fetal risk increases at doses above 1 g per day. See page 145	A newborn baby exhibited thrombocytopenia purpura, anemia that could have been drug-induced. Small amounts transfer into milk.
Valsartan antihypertensive	Angiotensive II receptor antagonists may cause fetal renal insufficiency, oligohydramnion, and hypocalvaria in late pregnancy, skull defects and fetal death. See pages 198, 204	No human data. Proposed monitoring: blood pressure. Advantages of breastfeeding should be considered.

(Continued)

	Pregnancy risk-benefit	Breastfeeding
Vancomycin antibiotic	No apparent malformation risk based on small numbers. Recommend Level 2 ultrasound in women exposed in T1.	No neonatal safety data. Proposed monitoring: diarrhea, due to potential change in gut flora. Advantages of breastfeeding should be considered.
Vecuroniun neuromuscular blocking agent	Limited first trimester reported experience. No apparent risk later in pregnancy based on small numbers.	No human data. Proposed monitoring: paresis, paralysis. Advantages of breastfeeding should be considered.
Venlafaxine antidepressant	No apparent malformation risk based on small numbers. No apparent neurobehavioral risk. At term—neonatal poor adaptation syndrome may occur. See pages 290, 293, 297	No apparent neonatal risk based on small numbers. Advantages of breastfeeding should be considered.
Verapamil antiarrhythmic	No apparent malformation risk based on small numbers.	No neonatal safety data. Proposed monitoring: heart rhythm.
Vinblastine anticancer	Cancer drugs inhibit cell division and proliferation and may cause birth defects in first trimester.	The infant should not be exposed to cancer drugs through milk.
Vincristine anticancer	Cancer drugs inhibit cell division and proliferation and may cause birth defects.	The infant should not be exposed to cancer drugs through milk.

(*Continued*)

	Pregnancy risk-benefit	Breastfeeding
Vitamins	A: May be associated with neural tube defects when dose is in access of 8000 IU per day.	No apparent neonatal risk.
	B: No apparent fetal risks at recommended daily allowance (RDA).	No apparent neonatal risk.
	C: No apparent fetal risk at RDA.	No apparent neonatal risk.
	D: No apparent fetal risk at RDA.	No apparent neonatal risk.
	E: No apparent fetal risk at RDA. See pages 218, 221	No apparent neonatal risk.
Zafirlukast antiasthma	No human data. There are leukotriene receptor antagonists with wider record of fetal safety (i.e., Montelukost)	No neonatal safety data. Advantages of breastfeeding should be considered.
Zalcitabine anti-HIV	No apparent malformation risk based on small numbers. See page 312	HIV may be transferred to infant through breast milk.
Zanamivir antiviral	No human data. See page 312	No human data. Unlikely to appear in milk. Advantages of breastfeeding should be considered.
Zidovudine anti-HIV	No apparent fetal malformation or neurocognitive risks based on several studies and relatively large number. See page 312	HIV may be transferred to the infant through breast milk.

(Continued)

	Pregnancy risk-benefit	Breastfeeding
Zolmitriptan antimigraine	No human data. There are safety data on other members of this class (e.g., sumatriptan)	No human data. Advantages of breastfeeding should be considered.
Zolpidem hypnotic	No apparent malformation risk based on small numbers.	No neonatal safety data. Minimal levels in milk. Proposed monitoring: CNS depression. Advantages of breastfeeding should be considered.

SELECTED DRUGS, CHEMICALS, AND MEDICAL CONDITIONS: FREQUENTLY ASKED QUESTIONS WITH CONCISE EVIDENCE-BASED ANSWERS

CHAPTER 6

SAFE USE OF VALPROIC ACID DURING PREGNANCY

Gideon Koren, MD, FRCPC
Debra Kennedy, MBBS, FRACP

QUESTION

I have an epileptic patient who plans pregnancy. It took us years to control her seizures, and valproic acid seems to be the only way to control them. What is the risk to her fetus?

Answer

Neural tube defects (NTDs) are the most common of the major anomalies associated with in utero exposure to valproic acid. About 1% to 2% of exposed fetuses suffer adverse effects. The drug can also cause limb and cardiac malformation.

While NTDs are the more common malformations currently confirmed with valproic acid, other potential teratogenic effects, including facial dysmorphism, congenital cardiac defects, limb-reduction defects, and other skeletal anomalies, have been documented. Prenatal diagnosis, in particular maternal serum α-fetoprotein (AFP) screening and targeted ultrasonography, should be offered to all pregnant women exposed to valproic acid, and couples need to be made aware of the prenatal diagnostic options available to them. Periconceptional prophylaxis with high-dose folic acid has also been recommended for all women receiving valproic acid, although it was not effective in animals and counseling should emphasize pregnancy planning to optimize folic acid supplementation.

In addition to being a first-line drug for epilepsy, valproic acid, a well-established anticonvulsant drug, is being used increasingly for managing conditions other than epilepsy, particularly bipolar and other affective disorders. Because of the demographics of the population affected by such

145

psychiatric conditions, a growing number of women of childbearing age are likely to be exposed to this teratogenic drug.

Neural tube defects, the most common of the major anomalies associated with in utero exposure to valproic acid, are estimated to occur in 1% to 2% of exposed fetuses.[1] Use of valproic acid appears to be associated specifically with lumbosacral meningomyeloceles rather than with other forms of NTD, such as anencephaly[2]: the ratio of meningomyelocele to anencephaly is reported in one series as being 33 to 1.[3] Valproic acid seems to predominantly affect closure site 5 (lumbosacral region) and to influence the process of canalization in forming the caudal end of the neural tube.[4] Carbamazepine, the other anticonvulsant drug known to be associated with increased risk of NTDs, does not appear to affect closure sites 5 and 1 preferentially, and meroacrania, holoacrania, and spina bifida cystica have all been reported in carbamazepine-exposed fetuses.[5]

In some cases, including the two cases reported in the series of Ardinger et al.,[6] the defects are low-lying lumbosacral lesions and might be covered with skin.

NEONATAL EFFECTS

Manifestations of withdrawal symptoms, including irritability, jitteriness, abnormal tone, feeding difficulties, and seizures, have also been described in infants of women using valproic acid during pregnancy (especially those receiving high doses in the last trimester of pregnancy).[7] Other neonatal consequences of maternal valproic acid use include hyperbilirubinemia, hepatotoxicity (sometimes fatal), transient hyperglycinemia, and intrauterine growth retardation.

PRENATAL ISSUES

Because NTDs are the most common, major malformations associated with valproic acid exposure, prenatal diagnosis is focused on their detection. The two main tools for prenatal detection of NTDs are AFP estimation and ultrasonography.

α-Fetoprotein   α-Fetoprotein is a glycoprotein produced initially by the yolk sac and then by the fetal liver and gastrointestinal tract. α-Fetoprotein can be measured in amniotic fluid and in maternal serum and is now used widely as a marker in prenatal maternal serum screening programs. In 1972, Brock and Sutcliff[8] demonstrated that pregnancies affected with open (not skin-covered) NTDs had high levels of AFP in the amniotic fluid. Because AFP is detectable in maternal serum, these estimations can also be used as screening tests for presence of open NTDs.

Targeted ultrasound Because skin-covered lesions might not be associated with raised AFP levels, accurate prenatal diagnosis of valproic acid associated NTDs is difficult. Prenatal evaluation of valproic acid exposed fetuses must, therefore, include targeted ultrasound examination, particularly of the caudal spine, even when AFP levels are normal.[9–11] Detailed ultrasound is effective in detecting limb anomalies and some cardiac malformation. Echocardiogram can further rule out the latter.

More subtle counseling issues are also raised because the neurologic deficits associated with such caudal lesions could be small. The main derangement could be bladder or bowel dysfunction, which would mean those affected are likely to be ambulatory and are unlikely to develop hydrocephalus.

Amniocentesis Amniocentesis can be offered to women as a somewhat more accurate measure of AFP levels than maternal serum testing, although clearly there are increased risks associated with this invasive procedure. Generally, amniocentesis is used when satisfactory ultrasound examination is not possible, for example, in extremely obese women. Another method for detecting NTDs is measuring acetylcholinesterase (AChE) in amniotic fluid, a somewhat more specific marker for NTDs than AFP levels.[12] When a mother's AFP level is elevated and results of ultrasound examination are normal, amniocentesis might be offered for more definitive diagnosis of NTDs through measuring levels of AFP and AChE in amniotic fluid.

Folic acid prophylaxis Prophylaxis with folic acid at a dose of 5 mg/day is recommended for all women planning pregnancy who are receiving valproic acid (or carbamazepine). Despite inconclusive results of animal studies and the lack of human studies showing that folic acid protects against valproic acid induced embryotoxicity and specifically NTDs, current clinical practice is still to recommend periconceptional supplementation with high-dose (4 to 5 mg/day) folic acid.

Concerns have been raised in the past that folic acid, particularly in large doses, could result in decreased absorption of zinc from the gastrointestinal tract. This could have serious clinical consequences in that zinc deficiency in animals has been reported to cause malformations, particularly of the central nervous system.[13] Dietary supplementation with 10 to 20 times the daily requirement of folic acid in rodents failed to decrease the embryotoxicity of valproic acid and had no effect on zinc levels in the maternal liver, brain, or kidney, or in embryonic tissues.[14]

Ideally, folic acid should be taken periconceptionally so that it is being taken at the critical time of neural tube closure (up to 5 weeks after conception). Women taking valproic acid should be counseled and strongly encouraged to plan their pregnancies so that they can begin taking folic acid once they stop using contraception.

REFERENCES

1. Koren G, Pastuszak AP, Ito S. Drugs in pregnancy. *N Engl J Med* 1998;338:1128–1137.
2. Lindhout D, Schmidt D. In-utero exposure to valproate and neural tube defects [letter]. *Lancet* 1986;1(8494):1392–1393.
3. Lindhout D, Omtzigt JG, Cornel MC. Spectrum of neural-tube defects in 34 infants prenatally exposed to antiepileptic drugs. *Neurology* 1992; 42(4 Suppl 5):111–118.
4. Van Allen MI, Kalousek DK, Chernoff GF, et al. Evidence for multi-site closure of the neural tube in humans. *Am J Med Genet* 1993;47: 723–743.
5. Rosa FW. Spina bifida in infants of women treated with carbamazepine during pregnancy. *N Engl J Med* 1991;324:674–677.
6. Ardinger HH, Atkin JF, Blackston RD, et al. Verification of the fetal valproate syndrome phenotype [review]. *Am J Med Genet* 1988;29:171–185.
7. Boussemart T, Bonneau D, Levard G, et al. Omphalocele in a newborn baby exposed to sodium valproate in utero. *Eur J Pediatr* 1995;154(3): 220–221.
8. Brock DGH, Sutcliff RC. Alphafetoprotein in the antenatal diagnosis of anencephaly and spina bifida. *Lancet* 1972;2:197–199.
9. Wladimiroff JW, Stewart PA, Reuss A, et al. The role of ultrasound in the early diagnosis of fetal structural defects following maternal anticonvulsant therapy. *Ultrasound Med Biol* 1988;14(8):657–660.
10. Weinbaum PJ, Cassidy SB, Vintzileos AM, et al. Prenatal detection of a neural tube defect after fetal exposure to valproic acid. *Obstet Gynecol* 1986;67(Suppl 3):S31–S33.
11. Guibaud S, Simplot A, Boisson C, et al. Prenatal diagnosis of 4 cases of spina bifida in mothers treated with valproate [in French]. *J Genet Hum* 1987;35(4):231–235.

12. Brock DJH, Barron L, van Heyningen V. Prenatal diagnosis of neural tube defects with a monoclonal antibody specific for acetylcholinesterase. *Lancet* 1985;2:5–8.
13. Keen CL, Hurley LS. Zinc and reproduction: effects of deficiency on fetal and postnatal development. In: Mills CF, ed. Zinc in human biology. New York, NY: *Springer-Verlag*; 1989. p. 83–92.
14. Hansen DK, Grafton TF, Dial SL, et al. Effect of supplemental folic acid on valproic acid-induced embryotoxicity and tissue zinc levels in vivo. *Teratology* 1995;2:277–285.

CHAPTER 7

CANCER CHEMOTHERAPY DURING PREGNANCY: CONSORTIUM OF CANCER IN PREGNANCY EVIDENCE

Michael Lishner, MD
Gideon Koren, MD, FRCPC

QUESTION

I have an 8 weeks' pregnant patient who was diagnosed with stage III Hodgkin's disease last week. The oncologist suggests delaying chemotherapy until the second trimester. What are the effects of chemotherapy on a fetus after the first trimester? Where can I find reliable information on the subject?

Answer

Available data suggest that exposure to chemotherapy during the first trimester of pregnancy is associated with increased risk of major malformations. Exposure during the second and third trimesters does not result in major malformations, but could have nonteratogenic effects, such as low birth weight. The brain develops throughout pregnancy, and it could be affected later in pregnancy.

Diagnosis of cancer during pregnancy is one of the most extreme scenarios in medicine: the creation of a new life might coincide with the mother's death. This situation can put immense stress on pregnant patients, their families, and medical staff. Cancer occurs only rarely during pregnancy; incidence is 0.07% to 0.1%.[1] The current trend to defer pregnancy until later in life might lead to increased incidence of cancer during pregnancy. There is, however, very little information on the effect of pregnancy on cancer and the effects of cancer and its therapy on pregnancy outcome.[2,3] Because chemotherapeutic agents in current use have substantially increased longevity and survival, it is important that physicians ensure optimal treatment for mothers without harming their fetuses.

Most chemotherapeutic agents have been shown to damage rapidly dividing cells, such as bone marrow, intestinal epithelium, and reproductive organs. Animal studies suggest that a fetus would be similarly affected by these agents because fetal tissues have a high growth rate. This damage could result in spontaneous abortions or malformations.[4]

Chemotherapeutic drugs are potent teratogens. Currently, there is very little information on the effect of cancer chemotherapy on human fetus.[5] The risk of malformations when chemotherapy is administered during the first trimester has been estimated at 10% for single-agent chemotherapy and at 25% for combination chemotherapy.[6,7] Thus, chemotherapeutic agents should be avoided during the first trimester.

There is no evidence of increased risk of teratogenesis during the second and third trimesters.[5] A recent report on a small series of breast cancer patients confirmed, prospectively, that chemotherapy is effective and safe when administered after the first trimester.[8] The long-term nonteratogenic effects of chemotherapy remain largely unknown. There have been reports of increased risk of stillbirth, low birth weight, and intrauterine growth retardation following treatment in the second and third trimesters.[5,9]

When chemotherapy is administered during pregnancy, delivery of the infant should be timed to avoid the worst chemotherapy adverse effects (i.e., on blood cells) and their associated problems. Only a few reports associate chemotherapy administered to a mother with hemopoietic depression in her infant. Hemopoietic depression is self-limiting, but it increases the risk of neonatal infection and hemorrhage.[10]

The very limited available information does not suggest that children born to mothers treated with chemotherapy during pregnancy have impaired mental or physical development or will be infertile.[11] Incidence of second malignancies in these children should be evaluated. To date, only a single case report describes the occurrence of multiple malignancies in the son of a patient with acute lymphocytic leukemia who was exposed in utero to cyclophosphamide and steroids. His twin sister was not affected.[12] Antineoplastic agents administered systemically might reach clinically significant levels in breast milk, so breastfeeding is contraindicated.[13,14]

Use of cytotoxic immunosuppressive drugs for disorders other than cancer is increasing rapidly. These drugs are currently used for rheumatic disorders (especially in young women), after organ transplantation, and for other conditions. When these medications are used for non-malignant conditions, they are used at lower doses than for treating tumours. Alkylating agents (mainly cyclophosphamide) and antimetabolites (6-mercaptopurine and azathioprine) are often used for these conditions.[15]

Although there are some controlled studies on the effects of chemotherapy on fetuses, most literature is based on either case reports or small, uncontrolled series. In an attempt to close the gap and overcome some of the difficulties faced by physicians taking care of pregnant women with cancer, Motherisk has established the Consortium of Cancer in Pregnancy Evidence (CCoPE), an international group of oncologists, obstetricians, pediatricians, pharmacologists, geneticists, and specialists in related fields. The CCoPE has developed up-to-date, evidence-based information on diagnosis, management, prognosis, and effect on fetal outcome of cancer during pregnancy. This information is available in a new section of the Motherisk website at *www.motherisk.org*.

REFERENCES

1. Sutcliffe SB. Treatment of neoplastic disease during pregnancy: maternal and fetal effects. *Clin Invest Med* 1985;8:333–338.
2. Koren G, Weiner L, Lishner M, et al. Cancer in pregnancy: identification of unanswered questions on maternal and fetal risk. *Obstet Gynecol Survey* 1990;45:509–514.
3. Antonelli NM, Dotters DJ, Katz VL, et al. Cancer in pregnancy: a review of the literature. *Obstet Gynecol Survey* 1996;51:125–142.
4. Sokal J, Lessmann EM. Effects of cancer chemotherapeutic agents on the human fetus. *JAMA* 1960;172:1765–1772.
5. Zemlickis D, Lishner M, Koren G. Review of fetal effects of cancer chemotherapeutic agents. In: Koren G, Lishner M, Farine D, eds. Cancer in pregnancy. *Cambridge, England*: Cambridge University Press; 1996. p. 168–180.
6. Doll DC, Ringenberg S, Yarbro YW. Management of cancer during pregnancy. *Arch Intern Med* 1988;48:2058–2064.
7. Nicholson HO. Cytotoxic drugs in pregnancy: review of reported cases. *J Obstet Gynaecol Br Commonw* 1968;75:307–312.

8. Berry DL, Theriault RL, Holmes FA, et al. Management of breast cancer during pregnancy using a standardized protocol. *J Clin Oncol* 1999;17: 855–861.

9. Zemlickis D, Lishner M, Degendrofer P, et al. Fetal outcome following in utero exposure to cancer chemotherapy: the Toronto study. *Arch Intern Med* 1992;152:573–576.

10. Blatt J, Milvihill JJ, Ziegler JL, et al. Pregnancy outcome following cancer chemotherapy. *Am J Med* 1980;39:828–832.

11. Aviles A, Diaz-Maqueo JC, Talavera A, et al. Growth and development of children of mothers treated with chemotherapy during pregnancy. Current status of 43 children. *Am J Hematol* 1991;136:243–248.

12. Zemlickis D, Lishner M, Erlich R, et al. Teratogenicity and carcinogenicity in a twin exposed in utero to cyclophosphamide. *Teratog Carcinog Mutagen* 1993;13:139–143.

13. Egan PC, Costanza ME, Dodion P, et al. Doxorubicin and cisplatin excretion into human milk. *Cancer Treat Rep* 1985;69:1387–1389.

14. De Vries EGE, Van Der Zee AGJ, Uges DRA, et al. Excretion of platinum into breast milk. *Lancet* 1989;1:497.

15. Ebert U, Loffler H, Kirch W. Cytotoxic therapy and pregnancy. *Pharmacol Ther* 1997;74:207–220.

CHAPTER 8

CORTICOSTEROIDS AND NONSTEROIDAL ANTI-INFLAMMATORY DRUGS (NSAIDS) DURING PREGNANCY

Gideon Koren, MD, FRCPC

QUESTION

I am following up a former preterm infant, born at 29 weeks gestation after premature labor. This infant had a relatively benign hospital course and when discharged was not thought to have any complications of prematurity. Despite this, at 1-year-old his neurologic examination is abnormal: head circumference is on the 3rd percentile for age (weight on the 25th percentile), and he has increased tone in his lower legs and a moderate developmental delay. His discharge letter indicated that he was exposed antenatally to many doses of dexamethasone. Could this have adversely influenced his neurologic outcome?

Answer

Antenatal steroids are proven therapy for preventing respiratory distress syndrome and decrease both morbidity and mortality associated with prematurity. Use of multiple doses of antenatal steroids might adversely affect neurologic outcome. There is insufficient evidence to support routine use of multiple doses of antenatal steroids when delivery of a preterm infant is anticipated, especially due to evidence of commulative fetal brain damage with repeated doses.

▨ QUESTION

I have a patient with rheumatoid arthritis who needs ASA or another NSAID for pain control. She is now pregnant and is afraid to continue medication. How should I advise her?

Answer

The patient should continue with ASA or another NSAID if clinically indicated. During the second half of pregnancy, her fetus should be monitored carefully. If high doses are needed, fetal ultrasound and echocardiography should be used to monitor amniotic fluid and patency of the fetal ductus arteriosus. During the last 2 weeks of a term pregnancy, the dose should be reduced as much as the patient's condition allows to reduce the risks of peripartum bleeding, neonatal hemorrhage, and persistent fetal circulation.

The fetal and the neonatal risks associated with using cyclooxygenase inhibitors, such as ASA and other NSAIDs, during late pregnancy are the topic of ongoing debate.[1] In fetuses and neonates, the cyclooxygenase products prostaglandin E_2 and I_2 are potent dilators of the ductus arteriosus and pulmonary resistance arteries. Treating animal fetuses with cyclooxygenase inhibitors leads to constriction of the ductus arteriosus and redistribution of blood flow in other fetal vascular beds.[2] This has led to concern that there might be a causal relationship between cyclooxygenase inhibitors, prenatal ductal closure, and postnatal development of persistent pulmonary hypertension of the newborn (PPHN).

However, the magnitude of the physiologic role of vasodilatory prostaglandins in maintaining human ductus arteriosus patency and in the perinatal transition of blood circulation has not been established.[3] The existence of a causal association between fetal exposure to cyclooxygenase inhibitors and the occurrence of PPHN also remains unproven.

Recently, Van Marter et al.[4] attempted to investigate the association between several potential antenatal risk factors and PPHN. Using a case-control approach and interviewing mothers, they found an apparent association between antenatal consumption of ASA or NSAIDs and the occurrence of PPHN. Based on this apparent association and a discussion indicating biologic plausibility, the authors concluded that ASA and NSAIDs contribute to PPHN and that consuming these drugs during pregnancy should be avoided. Case-control studies can be powerful epidemiologic tools for investigating suspected associations between fairly common antenatal exposures and rare pregnancy outcomes. This study design can be ineffective if the outcome of the pregnancy has an effect on the retrieval of risk factors that were present during the pregnancy. If risk factors are obtained through interviews, they are subject to recall bias, and this must be adequately addressed in the design of the study. Selection of an appropriate control group is of utmost importance because mothers of healthy babies are much more likely to forget and not report events perceived as minor than mothers of unhealthy babies.[5] Failure to address recall bias actively is likely to result in false-positive associations similar to the results of early studies investigating the association between ASA and congenital malformations. One state-of-the-art case-control study, therefore, selected mothers of children with different malformations from the index malformation as the control group.[6]

Van Marter et al.[4] address the problem of recall bias by stating that they "do not have compelling evidence that control mothers selectively underreported any exposure." Most of the reported exposures took place during the first trimester, many even during the first month of pregnancy (i.e., more than 6 months before the interview). At the time of exposure, many mothers were probably unaware of the pregnancy. The median number of tablets taken during the entire pregnancy was low (four for ASAs, eight for NSAIDs). Such brief and early exposures are easily forgotten by mothers of healthy babies and are likely to be reported more often by mothers of unhealthy newborns who try to remember "what went wrong?"

To causally link antenatal ASA and NSAID exposure to PPHN, the authors cite animal studies and case reports. However, unlike their own series, all these articles deal with exposures during late pregnancy. When evaluating biologic plausibility, it is important to understand that the effects of drugs on fetuses are highly dependent on the stage of fetal development and that they differ widely between first and third trimester.

Van Marter et al. indirectly acknowledge the irrelevance of their citations by speculating on how exposure during early pregnancy might have caused neonatal PPHN. They speculate that SAS and NSAIDs might alter the pulmonary vasculature during early pregnancy with effects not visible until birth or that first-trimester use might be associated with third-trimester use of the drugs. However, persistent effects of ASA or NSAIDs after discontinuing the drug during early pregnancy have not been described, and an association between first-trimester and last-trimester use is negated by authors' own data.

It is unfortunate that, based on a study with less than optimal design and with a lack of biologic plausibility, recommendations with possibly wide implications were made. With the data presented and the available evidence, the recommendation to avoid these drugs is more misleading than informative. It can lead to inadequate treatment of serious conditions during pregnancy, unnecessary fears after exposure, and perhaps even termination of otherwise wanted pregnancies.[7]

To date, no evidence indicates that first-trimester exposure to NSAIDs or ASA is associated with any adverse pregnancy outcome. As documented by studies evaluating low-dose ASA for treating preeclampsia, low-dose ASA appears to have no adverse effects on fetuses or neonates when given late in pregnancy.[8]

More controversial is the use of higher doses of NSAIDs in ASA during the second half of pregnancy. Fetal exposure to indomethacin during late pregnancy has been associated with constriction of the ductus arteriosus and oligohydramnios in utero and with a variety of neonatal diseases, such as patent ductus arteriosus, necrotizing enterocolitis, and respiratory distress syndrome.[9] However, intrauterine effects were usually reversible upon discontinuation of the drug and the incidence of neonatal diseases was unlikely to be increased if indomethacin was given for only 2 to 3 days. In fact, the Society of Obstetricians and Gynecologists of Canada considers the short-term treatment of preterm labour with indomethacin worth further study.[10]

A recent meta-analysis of case control studies suggests association between ASA and gastroschisis.[11] It is possibnle that this may be due to certain upper respiratory tract infection viruses for which ASA is given symptomatically.

We need more information about the safety of NSAIDs or higher doses of ASA during the second half of pregnancy. The various fetal risks associated with use of these drugs during various stages of pregnancy illustrate well the complexity of issues in reproductive toxicology.

REFERENCES

1. Merrill JD, Clyman RI, Norton ME. Indomethacin as a tocolytic agent: the controversy continues. *J Pediatr* 1994;124:734–736.
2. Coceani F, Olley PM. The control of cardiovascular shunts in the fetal and perinatal period. *Can J Physiol Pharmacol* 1988;66:1129–1134.

3. Hammerman C. Patent ductus arteriosus. Clinical relevance of prostaglandins and prostaglandin inhibitors in PDA pathophysiology and treatment. *Clin Perinatol* 1995;22:457–479

4. Van Marter LJ, Leviton A, Allred EN, et al. Persistent pulmonary hypertension of the newborn and smoking and aspirin and nonsteroidal antiinflammatory drug consumption during pregnancy. *Pediatrics* 1996;97:658–663.

5. Werler MM, Pober BR, Nelson K, et al. Reporting accuracy among mothers of malformed and nonmalformed infants. *Am J Epidemiol* 1989;129:15–21.

6. Werler MM, Mitchell AA, Shapiro S. The relation of aspirin use during the first trimester of pregnancy to congenital cardiac defects. *N Engl J Med* 1989;321:1639–1642.

7. Koren G, Bologa M, Pastuszak A. The way women perceive teratogenic risk. The decision to terminate pregnancy. In: Koren G, editor. *Maternal-fetal toxicology: a clinician's guide.* 2nd ed. New York, NY: Marcel Dekker, 1994:727–736.

8. CLASP collaborative group. Low dose aspirin in pregnancy and early childhood development: follow up of the collaborative low dose aspirin study in pregnancy. *Br J Obstet Gynaecol* 1995;102:861–868.

9. Briggs GG, Freeman RK, Yaffee SJ. *Drugs in pregnancy and lactation.* 4th ed. Baltimore, Md: Williams and Wilkins, 1994:443–452.

10. Hannah M, Amankwah K, Barrett J, et al. The Canadian consensus on the use of tocolytics for preterm labour. *J Soc Obstet Gynaecol Can* 1995;17:1089–1138.

CHAPTER 9

MATERNAL OBESITY AND PRENATAL RISK

Gideon Koren, MD, FRCPC

QUESTION

One of my patients is taking olanzapine for schizophrenia. She has gained a lot of weight, which, I understand, often happens with some of the new atypical antipsychotics. Due to her weight gain, she failed to notice she had become pregnant. Is she at risk?

Answer

Experience with olanzapine is relatively new, but available prospective data do not show increased teratogenic risk. Adiposity, on the other hand, is associated with increased risk of neural tube defects. Only some of this risk can be reduced by folate supplementation.

Obesity during pregnancy is associated with a long list of acknowledged health risks, including higher prevalence of cesarean section,[1] hypertension,[2] deep vein thrombosis,[3] and diabetes mellitus.[4] In addition, obesity is associated with a higher need for cesarian section. In this update, however, we will focus on the relatively unknown risk of neural tube defects (NTDs).

Several epidemiologic studies have suggested that being overweight before pregnancy is a risk factor for NTDs. A large case-control study of 604 fetuses or infants with NTDs, and 1658 fetuses or infants with other major malformations, showed that risk of NTDs increased from 1.9 (95% confidence interval [CI] 1.2 to 2.9) for women weighing 80 to 89 kg to 4.0 (95% CI 1.6 to 9.9) for women weighing 110 kg or more.[5] The reference group for comparison consisted of women weighing between 50 and 59 kg.

After controlling for folate intake, there was still a threefold higher risk of NTDs in the heaviest groups. Intake of 400 µg or more of folate reduced NTD risk by 40% among women weighing less than 70 kg, but did not decrease risk at all among heavier women. These results suggest that inadequate folate intake is not the mechanism leading to increased risk of NTDs among the babies of obese women.

It is now generally accepted that a body mass index >29 kg/m^2 doubles the risk of NTDs.[6] A recent study has shown that the elevated risk encompasses open or closed, isolated, nonisolated, high, low, or open/isolated/high phenotypes of spina bifida. Risk appears to be higher among female offspring.[7]

With the introduction of atypical antipsychotics, such as clozapine, olanzapine, and others, it will be important to ensure appropriate intake of folic acid to account for the increased body mass commonly associated with these medications.[8] Because many women taking these drugs become obese, it makes clinical sense to monitor them with ultrasound and α-fetoprotein to rule out NTDs. These patients should also be referred to high-risk perinatal programs for diagnosis and management of other complications related to weight gain (e.g., hypertension, diabetes, and deep vein thrombosis).

REFERENCES

1. Kaiser PS, Kirby RS. Obesity as a risk factor in a low-risk population. *Obstet Gynecol* 2001;97:39–43.
2. Broughton PF, Roberts JM. Hypertension in pregnancy. *J Hum Hypertens* 2000;14:705–724.
3. Samama MM. An epidemiologic study of risk factors for deep vein thrombosis in medical out-patients: the Sirius study. *Arch Intern Med* 2000;160: 3415–3420.
4. Moore LL, Singer MR, Bradlee ML, et al. A prospective study of the risk of congenital defects associated with maternal obesity and diabetes mellitus. *Epidemiology* 2000;11:689–694.
5. Werler MM, Louik C, Shapiro S, et al. Prepregnant weight in relation to risk of neural tube defects. *JAMA* 1996;275:1089–1092.
6. Shaw GM, Velie EM, Schaffer D. Risk of neural tube defect-affected pregnancies among obese women. *JAMA* 1996;275:1093–1096.
7. Shaw GM, Todoroff K, Finnell RH, Lammer EJ. Spina bifida phenotypes in infants or fetuses of obese mothers. *Teratology* 2000;61:376–381.
8. Karagianis J. Olanzapine and weight gain [letter]. *Can J Psychiatry* 2000; 45:493.

ANTIHISTAMINES ARE APPARENTLY SAFE DURING THE FIRST TRIMESTER

Gideon Koren, MD, FRCPC

QUESTION

One of my patients has just found out she is pregnant. This is allergy season, and she claims that she cannot function in her executive position at work without her antihistamines. How safe are antihistamines for her?

Answer

You can assure your patient that, based on a large number of studies, antihistamines do not appear to increase teratogenic risk.

During early pregnancy, a critical stage of organogenesis that might be adversely affected by drugs and environmental agents, women receive more prescriptions for antihistamines than for any other agent except vitamins.[1] Antihistamines are used during early pregnancy mainly to treat morning sickness.

Although antihistamines have been widely prescribed to large numbers of pregnant women, their safety has not been established unequivocally, and some studies have reported increased teratogenic risk. Removal of Bendectin (doxylamine-pyridoxine) from the American market by its manufacturer in 1983, because of the litigation surrounding it, highlights public sensitivity to potential teratogenic risk. Following removal of Bendectin, the most commonly used agent for morning sickness in the United States, rates of hospitalization due to hyperemesis gravidarum doubled, underscoring the serious consequences of wrongly perceiving a drug as a human teratogen when it is needed by large numbers of women.[2]

We have recently done a meta-analysis of all controlled studies of anti-histamine use in early pregnancy, in order to quantify the relative risk of major malformations associated with antihistamine use.[3] Twenty-four studies met our inclusion criteria; more than 200,000 women were involved. The summary odds ratio (OR) for major malformations in babies of women exposed to antihistamines during the first trimester was 0.76 (95% Confidence Interval (CI) 0.6 to 0.94).

About 60% of women experience nausea and vomiting during the first trimester, and about half of them are treated with antihistamines. Our analysis indicates no positive association between use of antihista-mines in the first trimester and rates of major malformations. An overall OR of 0.76 with a 95% CI of 0.6 to 0.94 indicates an apparent 24% protective effect. Proving that antihistamines do not have a teratogenic effect is of utmost importance, because many women and their physi-cians are reluctant to treat morning sickness effectively due to the per-ception of teratogenic risk. Our analysis, which included more than 200,000 women in 24 different studies, has an unprecedented power to reject the suggestion that antihistamines have teratogenic potential.

The suggestion that antihistamines have a protective effect against some major malformations has not been examined yet. Severe nausea and vomiting is often debilitating and occasionally life-threatening. It is conceivable that suboptimal maternal nutrition combined with dehydra-tion and electrolyte imbalances resulting from hyperemesis gravidarum create suboptimal conditions for embryonic growth. Animal studies have demonstrated that maternal nutritional deficiencies during gestation result in increased risk of malformations in offspring.[4] In humans, hyper-emesis gravidarum has been associated with increased risk of central nervous system malformations, and eye and ear malformations.[5] Hence, by preventing the untoward effects of nausea and vomiting, antihista-mines might have a protective effect. This possibility will have to be addressed by future research.

An alternative explanation is that pregnancies characterized by vom-iting are biologically different from those without vomiting, and those with vomiting have a better prognosis. The idea that vomiting signals better pregnancy outcome has been studied in the past,[6] but the studies did not specify which antiemetic drugs the women used.

In summary, pregnant women suffering from morning sickness and its consequences, or allergies, that do not respond to nonpharmaco-logic treatment can safely use antihistamines.

REFERENCES

1. Bonati M, Tognoni G. Drug use in pregnancy: a preliminary report of the International Co-operative Drug Utilization Study. *Pharm World Sci* 1990;12(2):75–78.
2. Skalnick A. Key witness against morning sickness drug faces scientific fraud charges. *JAMA* 1990;263:1468–1473.
3. Seto E, Einarson T, Koren G. Pregnancy outcome following first trimester exposure to antihistamines; a meta-analysis. *Am J Perinatol.* In press.
4. Warkany J, Petering H. Congenital malformations of the brain caused by short zinc deficiencies in rats. *Am J Ment Defic* 1973;77:645-653.
5. Depue RH, Bernstein L, Ross RK, et al. Hyperemesis gravidarum in relation to estradiol levels, pregnancy outcome, and other maternal factors: a sero-epidemiologic study. *Am J obstet gynecol* 1987; 156:1137–1141.
6. Brandes JM. First trimester nausea and vomiting as related to outcome of pregnancy. *Obstet Gynecol* 1967;30:427–431.

CHAPTER 11

CAFFEINE DURING PREGNANCY?: IN MODERATION

Gideon Koren, MD, FRCPC

QUESTION

Many of my female patients, those who plan pregnancy or have conceived, are afraid of any intake of caffeine. This often makes their lives miserable during pregnancy. Is this justified scientifically?

Answer

Motherisk's recent meta-analysis suggests that the risks for miscarriage and fetal growth retardation increase only with daily doses of caffeine above 150 mg/day, equivalent to 1.5 cups (250 mL/cup) of coffee a day. It is possible that some of this presumed risk is due to confounders, such as cigarette smoking.

In 1980, the U.S. Food and Drug Administration (FDA) issued a warning regarding use of caffeine during pregnancy.[1] Because conclusions about human teratogenicity could not be definite at that time, the FDA suggested that, as a precautionary measure, pregnant women should be advised to avoid or limit consumption of food or drugs containing caffeine. Due to the large worldwide consumption of caffeinated beverages (e.g., coffee, tea, cola), it is important to know whether such a warning is actually warranted. If caffeine consumption during pregnancy were linked to adverse effects, such as spontaneous abortion or fetal growth retardation, those findings would have important implications for public health. Furthermore, the potential effect of such an association is underscored by the fact that low birth weight is associated with high mortality and morbidity among neonates.

Caffeine clearance from the body continues essentially unchanged during the first trimester of pregnancy, but is substantially delayed during the second and third trimesters, because the half-life of caffeine extends to 10.5 hour from a normal of 2.5 hour to 4.5 hour.[2] Caffeine is known to cross the placenta readily; substantial quantities pass into the amniotic fluid and umbilical cord blood, and appear in the urine and plasma of neonates. In addition, human fetuses and neonates have low levels of the enzymes needed to metabolize caffeine.

Several mechanisms by which caffeine might produce adverse outcomes have been postulated. For example, caffeine increases cellular cyclic adenosine monophosphate (cAMP) through inhibition of phosphodiesterases. The rise in cAMP might interfere with fetal cell growth and development.[3]

ANIMAL STUDIES

Animal studies of caffeine and pregnancy outcomes have had varied results. Some studies have suggested a link between caffeine and teratogenesis, fetal resorption, and low fetal weight.[4,5] An increase in the rate of malformations, specifically cleft palate and ectrodactyly, was demonstrated in rats and mice given caffeine doses of 100 mg/kg/day or more.[5] This effect was not seen at doses of 50 mg/kg/day, and humans ingest caffeine at substantially lower doses of 1.7 to 4.5 mg/kg/day.[5]

Epidemiologic studies have produced incomplete or conflicting results concerning the effects of caffeine exposure during pregnancy. Motherisk recently conducted a meta-analysis to determine the association of moderate to heavy caffeine consumption during pregnancy with spontaneous abortion and fetal growth in humans.[6]

MOTHERISK'S META-ANALYSIS

For spontaneous abortion, five studies were included (three cohort and two case-control studies) involving a total of 42,889 patients. The combined odds ratio (OR) was 1.36 (95% confidence interval [CI] 1.29 to 1.45), indicating that mothers who consumed caffeine had a higher risk of spontaneous abortion than those who did not. For fetal growth, five studies involving a total of 64,268 patients were included. Combined relative risk was 1.51 (1.39 to 1.63). Risk ratio for comparing moderate caffeine consumption with controls (0 to 150 mg of caffeine consumption) was 1.33 (95% CI 1.21 to 1.47) and for comparing heavy caffeine consumption with controls was 1.81 (95% CI 1.61 to 2.04). A risk ratio of 1.06 (95% CI 1.00 to 1.13) resulted from comparing our controls with "zero" caffeine consumption;

because this risk ratio included unity, it validated our choice of control group. A recent study[7] where levels of the caffeine metabolite paraxanthine were correlated with risk of spontaneous abortion corroborated our analysis. It showed that only very excessive coffee consumption is associated with increased risk.

LIMITATIONS OF STUDIES

When combining studies addressing the reproductive risks of caffeine, we have to acknowledge the limitations inherent in this research. All studies accepted into the meta-analysis depended on mothers' or expectant mothers' recall of their level and sources of caffeine consumption. The ability to accurately recall and report the amount of caffeine ingested partly depends on whether subjects are questioned prospectively or retrospectively.

A second possible error introduced involves caffeine measurement. How did subjects estimate the amount of caffeine contained in specific servings? Most studies used an educated "guess" by taking the averages of various samples obtained from their study population and analyzed for content.

A third potential error in estimating caffeine intake involves not identifying all sources of caffeine consumed. Although coffee is the most common source of caffeine, failure to include other sources, such as chocolate and cola, would lead to a degree of underestimation of caffeine use. It is assumed that this underestimation would occur to the same extent in control and study groups.

Wilcox and associates[8] showed that approximately 25% of biochemically detected pregnancies ended before being clinically detected. We might assume that early spontaneous abortion would follow the patterns of late spontaneous abortion among the various stratifications of caffeine consumption. The extent to which this assumption is valid determines the amount of error introduced into the meta-analysis.

Various confounding factors were identified in the articles Motherisk accepted. The most important common confounders appear to be concurrent smoking, alcohol use, maternal age over 35, and previous spontaneous abortion. Most other confounding factors would be equally distributed among the various stratifications of caffeine consumption. Levels of smoking, alcohol use, and maternal age, however, have been shown to be positively correlated with levels of caffeine consumption.[9]

Risk of spontaneous abortion increases as the quantity of cigarettes smoked per day increases.[9] In most of the five studies in the main analysis for spontaneous abortion, the ORs did not change significantly even after researchers adjusted for smoking and other confounders (as reported in each study).

Our results suggest a small but statistically significant increase in risk of spontaneous abortion and low-birth-weight babies in pregnant women consuming more than 150 mg of caffeine per day. Pregnant women should be encouraged to be aware of dietary caffeine intake and to consume less than 150 mg of caffeine a day from all sources throughout pregnancy.

REFERENCES

1. Caffeine and pregnancy. *US Food and Drug Administration Drug Bull* 1980;10(3):19–20.
2. Knutti R, Rothweiler H, Schlatter C. The effect of pregnancy on the pharmacokinetics of caffeine. *Arch Toxicol Suppl* 1982;5 (Suppl):187–192.
3. Weathersbee PS, Lodge R. Caffeine: its direct and indirect influence on reproduction. *J Reprod Med* 1977;19:55–63.
4. Thayer PS, Palm PE. A current assessment of the mutagenic and teratogenic effects of caffeine. *CRC Crit Rev Toxicol* 1975;3:345–369.
5. Wilson JG, Scott WJ. The teratogenic potential of caffeine in laboratory animals. In: Dews PB, ed. *Caffeine: perspectives from recent research.* Berlin, *Ger: Springer-Verlag*; 1984:165–187.
6. Fernandes O, Shabarwal M, Smiley T, et al. Moderate to heavy caffeine consumption and relationship to spontaneous abortion and abnormal fetal growth: a meta-analysis. *Reprod Toxicol* 1998;12:435–444.
7. Klebanoff MA, Levine RJ, Der Sinonian R, et al. Maternal serum paraxantine, a caffeine metabolite, and the risk of spontaneous abortion. *N Engl J Med* 1999;34:1639–1644.
8. Wilcox AJ, Weinberg CR, Baird DD. Risk factors for early pregnancy loss. *Epidemiology* 1990;1:382–385.
9. Golding J. Reproduction and caffeine consumptionóa literature review. *Early Hum Dev* 1995;43:1–14.

CHAPTER 12

ANTIMALARIAL DRUGS FOR RHEUMATOID DISEASE DURING PREGNANCY

Gideon Koren, MD, FRCPC

QUESTION

One of my patients, who has rheumatoid arthritis, has just found out she is pregnant. She is being treated with hydroxychloroquine. I could not find anything about the safety of this drug during pregnancy.

ANSWER

Most of the literature on this drug relates to prophylaxis for malaria. Much lower doses than those used for rheumatic diseases are given for malaria prophylaxis with no adverse fetal effects. Several studies on use of the drug for rheumatic diseases during pregnancy also failed to show adverse fetal effects, although, in most cases, only first-trimester exposure was reported.

Chloroquine and hydroxychloroquine have been shown effective for rheumatoid arthritis; they compare favorably with gold therapy early in the disease.[1] They have an advantage over gold in that they are given by mouth once a day and do not have the renal and hematologic complications of gold therapy. These antimalarial drugs have been shown beneficial for treating some forms of skin rash as well as systemic symptoms associated with systemic lupus erythematosus (SLE).[2] Antimalarials have also been shown to be effective for treating psoriatic arthritis.[3]

For adults, the main toxicity of antimalarial drugs is gastrointestinal irritation and the eye damage that results from their deposition in the retina. This appears to be dose related and is usually reversible, although there have been reports of persistent retinopathy.[4] In virtually all cases, some chloroquine is deposited in the cornea, which is of minor clinical importance and does not correlate with retinal deposits. Corneal deposits are not a contraindication to antimalarial therapy. Regular ophthalmologic examinations are recommended to detect early retinal toxicity, and antimalarial therapy should be stopped if evidence of retinal toxicity is found. Hydroxychloroquine is reported to be associated with less toxicity than chloroquine sulfate.

The main concern for a fetus is the effect of antimalarial drugs on retinal development, development of thrombocytopenia, and central nervous system abnormalities (ototoxicity has been reported sporadically after use of chloroquine during pregnancy[4]). Most of the data on use of antimalarial drugs during pregnancy relate to prophylaxis for malaria, where much lower doses than those used for rheumatic diseases are prescribed. The drugs have been used inadvertently during the first trimester with no adverse effects in some patients with SLE.[5,6] Although some patients treated with antimalarials are reported to have uncomplicated pregnancies, we cannot recommend use of these drugs for pregnant patients with rheumatic diseases throughout pregnancy because available data on the safety of high doses relate only to first-trimester exposure.

Although use of chloroquine and hydroxychloroquine to prevent malaria is probably safe during pregnancy, use of much higher doses for treating SLE and rheumatoid arthritis during pregnancy is controversial. We analyzed the cases of 24 pregnant women with a total of 27 pregnancies who had taken these drugs during the first trimester.[6] Chloroquine and hydroxychloroquine were given to 11 patients with SLE, 3 with rheumatoid arthritis, and 4 for malaria prophylaxis. Most of these women had already been taking antimalarial drugs for between 1 and 172 months before pregnancy (mean, 32.2 months).

Of the 27 pregnancies, 14 resulted in normal full-term babies, 6 were aborted due to severe disease or social conditions, 3 were stillbirths, and 4 resulted in spontaneous abortions. No congenital abnormalities were detected in the 14 live births between ages 9 months and 19 years (mean, 5.3 years). All these children are physically and developmentally normal with no clinical evidence of eye or ear defects. The 7 pregnancies associated with fetal loss occurred mainly among patients with active SLE, although patients with rheumatoid arthritis and 2 of the patients treated prophylactically for malaria had stillbirths and spontaneous abortions.

Among 215 pregnancies reported exposed to chloroquine and hydroxychloroquine, including those in our study, only 7 (3.3%) had congenital abnormalities. The risk associated with antimalarial drugs might be cumulative; further studies are needed to clarify the safety of this drug later in pregnancy.

Hydroxychloroquine is found in human milk, but infants would be exposed to only 2% of the maternal dose/kg daily and, therefore, breastfeeding is not contraindicated.[7]

REFERENCES

1. Rynes RI. Antimalarial drugs. In: Kelley WN, Harris ED, Ruddy S, Sledge CB, editors. *Textbook of rheumatology.* 4th ed. Philadelphia, Pa: WB Saunders; 1993. p. 731–742.
2. Esdaile JM. The efficacy of antimalarials in systemic lupus erythematosus. *Lupus* 1993;2(Suppl 1):S3–S8.
3. Gladman DD, Blake R, Brubacher B, et al. Chloroquine therapy in psoriatic arthritis. *J Rheumatol* 1992;19:1724–1726.
4. Hart CW, Nauton RF. The ototoxicity of chloroquine phosphate. *Arch Otolaryngol* 1964;80:497–512.
5. Tozman ECS, Urowitz MB, Gladman DD. Systemic lupus erythematosus and pregnancy. *J Rheumatol* 1980;7:624–632.
6. Levy M, Buskila D, Gladman DD. Pregnancy outcome following first trimester exposure to chloroquine. *Am J Perinatol* 1991;8:174–177.
7. Nation RL, Hacektt LP, Dusci LJ, et al. Excretion of hydroxychloroquine in human milk. *Br J Clin Pharmacol* 1984;17:368–369.

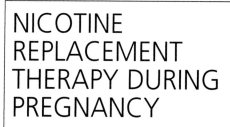

CHAPTER 13

NICOTINE REPLACEMENT THERAPY DURING PREGNANCY

Gideon Koren, MD

QUESTION

Several years ago you argued in favor of trying nicotine replacement therapy during pregnancy. The Ontario Medical Association recommended the same. Are there any studies now to show that the patch works?

ANSWER

A large randomized, blinded study from Denmark has shown that the rate of quitting smoking during pregnancy using the nicotine patch is very low and not different from the rate among those given placebo. Preliminary data suggest that women who cannot quit smoking after the first trimester metabolize nicotine rapidly and that this could be a mechanism for their failure to quit.

An estimated 25% to 30% of women smoke cigarettes at the beginning of pregnancy.[1] While some of them succeed in quitting smoking, many are unable to do so. While many psychosocial factors affect smoking patterns, it is now widely recognized that the inability to stop smoking cigarettes is due to dependence on nicotine. Studies of nicotine replacement therapy (NRT) show that nicotine patches, gum, or intranasal preparations are superior to placebo in helping people quit.[2]

Concerns about using NRT during pregnancy stem from the observed teratogenicity of nicotine itself in animals.[3] Motherisk has shown that physicians can monitor nicotine serum levels in pregnant women using the patch and thus ensure their concentrations do not exceed levels encountered during smoking.[4]

A recent study by a Danish group reported on the first randomized placebo-controlled study of NRT in pregnant women: 124 women were randomized to receive the nicotine patch and 126 to receive placebo. All participating women could not quit smoking during the first trimester of pregnancy. They smoked 10 or more cigarettes daily and were less than 22 weeks pregnant. Both groups received counseling during the study.[5] Compliance with the assigned treatment was low in both groups: 83% of the nicotine group and 92% of the placebo group did not use all their patches. Three months postpartum only 20% of the women in both groups were not smoking. Why are results of NRT so disappointing among pregnant women? Why are they not achieving better smoking cessation rates than with placebo?

During the first trimester of pregnancy, many women quit smoking. Hence, those who cannot quit and who opt to try NRT are a highly selected group. In Motherisk's experience, women who ask to receive NRT started smoking at a mean age of 12 years (some were as young as 9), smoked an average of 24 cigarettes a day, did not reduce cigarette consumption during pregnancy, and in most cases, lit their first cigarette within 5 minutes of waking up.[6]

Most of these women's partners were also smoking, and they had made many attempts to quit the habit. It is interesting that their serum levels of nicotine were lower than expected while their concentrations of the oxidative metabolite, cotinine, were higher than expected. This could mean that these women tend to be rapid metabolizers of nicotine, which would engender a greater need to consume more cigarettes, which in turn would prevent them from stopping smoking even with the motivation created by pregnancy.[6]

Should we abandon using NRT during pregnancy? Probably not. Perhaps these women need more intense therapy than the therapy used in the Danish study. In a much smaller study than the Danish one, the Motherisk team had three successes among 18 women who received NRT compared with none among the placebo group.[7] It is possible that, because they are rapid metabolizers of nicotine, pregnant women need higher doses of nicotine in the patch than those given to non-pregnant women. Also, the counseling in our study seem to be more intensive than that described in the Danish trial.

As with any therapeutic trial, the Danish study will have to be repeated to ensure generalizability of results. The set might not be over, but it appears that placebo has won the first game.

REFERENCES

1. Gilles P, Wakefield M. Smoking in pregnancy. *Curr Obstet Gynecol* 1993;3: 157–161.
2. Benowitz NL. The use of pharmacotherapies for smoking cessation during pregnancy. *Tobacco Control* 2000;9(Suppl 3):91–94.
3. Slotkin TA. Fetal nicotine or cocaine exposure: which one is worse? *J Pharmacol Exp Ther* 1998;285:931–945.
4. Hackman R, Kapur B, Koren G. Use of the nicotine patch by pregnant women. *N Engl J Med* 1999;341:1700.
5. Wisborg K, Henriksen TB, Jespersen LB, et al. Nicotine patches for pregnant smokers: a randomized controlled study. *Obstet Gynecol* 2000;96: 967–971.
6. Selby P, Kapur B, Hackman R, et al. Women who cannot quit smoking during pregnancy: a possible pharmacokinetic predisposition. *Ther Drug Monit.* In press.
7. Kapur B, Hackman R, Selby P, et al. A randomized double-blind placebo control trial of nicotine replacement therapy in pregnancy. *Curr Ther Res. lin Exp* In press.

SAFETY OF COLCHICINE THERAPY DURING PREGNANCY

Ran D. Goldman, MD
Gideon Koren, MD, FRCPC

QUESTION

A 27-year-old patient in our clinic with familial Mediterranean fever (FMF) has been treated with colchicine for the last decade. She is planning her first pregnancy. What recommendations should we give her regarding use of colchicine before and during pregnancy, bearing in mind that discontinuation of colchicine could lead to complications from amyloidosis?

Answer

Colchicine passes through the placenta in humans, is teratogenic in animals, and raises rates of male and female infertility. Based on several patients with chromosomal anomalies, some authorities recommend that patients who require colchicine therapy during pregnancy undergo amniocentesis with karyotyping. In contrast, an increasing body of evidence suggests that colchicine use throughout pregnancy carries no substantial teratogenic or mutagenic risk when used at recommended doses. Its use prevents febrile attacks of FMF and reduces the frequency of renal complications.

Colchicine, a microtubule growth inhibitor, affects mitosis and other microtubule-dependent functions of cells, including the phagocytic properties of polymorphonuclear cells. As a therapeutic agent, the drug has relatively few approved indications.[1] While FMF is the most common indication for colchicine therapy,[2] colchicine has long been used to prevent or mitigate acute and chronic gout. Less frequently, colchicine is used for treating liver cirrhosis; biliary cirrhosis; and certain skin disorders, such as psoriasis, palmoplantar pustulosis, Behçet's disease, dermatitis herpetiformis, scleroderma, and condyloma acuminatum.

Familial Mediterranean fever is an autosomal recessive disease that primarily affects people of Jewish, Armenian, Arabic, and Turkish ancestry.[3] About half the patients affected have symptoms in their first decade of life; only 5% of patients develop FMF after the age of 30.[4] The disease manifests clinically by recurrent attacks of fever, peritonitis, pleuritis, arthritis, or erysipelas-like skin findings. Attacks, which generally last 1 to 4 days and occur every 3 to 4 months, are triggered by such factors as physical and emotional stress, menstruation, and a high-fat diet.[5] Between attacks, patients are healthy and usually free of symptoms.

Colchicine was introduced in the early 1970s to prevent and decrease the severity of FMF attacks.[6] Its anti-inflammatory properties made it a good therapeutic candidate, and up to 90% of patients had marked reduction or complete remission of symptoms during continuous treatment.[7-9] Because colchicine is teratogenic in animals[1] and passes through the placenta in humans,[10] it was contraindicated during pregnancy before the 1990s.

EFFECT ON FERTILITY

Colchicine was thought to affect fertility. Ehrenfeld et al.[9] reported periods of infertility in 13 of 36 women with FMF taking long-term colchicine treatment (prevention of human cytotrophoblast differentiation into syncytiotrophoblasts following in vitro colchicine treatment suggested a possible mechanism for female infertility[11]). Azoospermia or impaired sperm penetration were found in 20% of men taking colchicine,[12] although the inconsistent sperm pathologies could be explained by variability in disease pathophysiology rather than by colchicine's effect on sperm production or function.[13] To date, no clear link between infertility and colchicine has been established.

RISK OR BENEFIT?

Even with these tentative risks of teratogenicity and infertility, discontinuing colchicine treatment before or during pregnancy appears to carry greater risk than maintaining it. Amyloidosis is the main complication of untreated FMF, and the resulting nephropathy[1] has been correlated with adverse maternal and fetal outcomes.[14] Evidence indicates that colchicine protects against amyloidosis in patients with FMF.[15] Proteinuria was found in 4 of 960 (0.42%) patients compliant with colchicine treatment compared with 16 of 54 (29.6%) noncompliant patients in a study of 1070 patients followed for 4 to 11 years. Results of another study indicated that colchicine increased survival of those with primary amyloidosis.[16] It is possible that pregnancy exacerbates amyloid nephropathy in patients with FMF.[17]

Several case reports support the safety of colchicine during pregnancy. Zemer et al.[18] reported on three pregnant FMF-affected sisters. Two discontinued colchicine therapy during pregnancy and had subsequent nephropathy, amyloidosis, and febrile episodes; one of these two died within 2 years from end-stage renal failure. Nevertheless, both had delivered healthy children. The third sister continued colchicine therapy throughout pregnancy and had a healthy child with no reported complications. Two other pregnancies in FMF patients, complicated by ascites and amyloidosis, have ended successfully under continuous colchicine treatment.[19]

A successful pregnancy of a colchicine-treated FMF patient induced by in vitro fertilization[20] has been reported, and retrospective studies corroborate colchicine's safety during pregnancy. Among 84 colchicine-treated patients, 3 men and 7 women had healthy children. One pregnancy ended in spontaneous abortion, possibly as a result of noncompliance with colchicine treatment and subsequent nephrotic amyloidosis.[21] Another review of 28 pregnancies in 36 FMF-affected women receiving long-term colchicine therapy[9] reported 16 healthy infants. Several other pregnancies ended in miscarriages at a rate similar to that in untreated FMF patients.

In a review of 116 colchicine-treated mothers with 225 pregnancies,[22] 40 were treated during the first trimester, 91 were treated to term, and 94 were untreated. Neither the colchicine-treated mothers nor their children were found to be adversely affected during 10 years of follow up.

Spontaneous abortions were more prevalent in the untreated group (20.2%) than the treated group (12.2%), an outcome possibly related to attacks of fever and peritoneal irritation in untreated FMF patients.

CONCLUSION

Current evidence supports the safety of colchicine use throughout pregnancy at recommended doses. Discontinuing the drug during pregnancy might be detrimental for a woman with FMF. As yet, colchicine's link to infertility has not been fully established. Use of colchicine during pregnancy for gout and other diseases is not well documented, and risks of teratogenicity cannot be completely ruled out. If colchicine is to be used during pregnancy, caution should be exercised, and amniocentesis with karyotyping[9] should be considered due to the mutagenic risk shown in animals.

REFERENCES

1. Levy M, Spino M, Read SE. Colchicine: a state-of-the-art review. *Pharmacotherapy* 1991;11(3):196–211.
2. Ostensen M, Ramsey-Goldman R. Treatment of inflammatory rheumatic disorders in pregnancy: what are the safest treatment options? *Drug Saf* 1998;19:389–410.
3. Balow JE Jr, Shelton DA, Orsborn A, et al. A high-resolution genetic map of the familial Mediterranean fever candidate region allows identification of haplotype-sharing among ethnic groups. *Genomics* 1997;44:280–291.
4. Sohar E, Gafni J, Pras M, et al. Familial Mediterranean fever. A survey of 470 cases and review of the literature. *Am J Med* 1967;43:227–253.
5. Ben-Chetrit E, Levy M. Familial Mediterranean fever. *Lancet* 1998;351: 659–664.
6. Goldfinger SE. Colchicine for familial Mediterranean fever. *N Engl J Med* 1972;287:1302.
7. Zemer D, Revach M, Pras M, et al. A controlled trial of colchicine in preventing attacks of familial Mediterranean fever. *N Engl J Med* 1974;291: 932–934.
8. Dinarello CA, Wolff SM, Goldfinger SE, et al. Colchicine therapy for familial Mediterranean fever. A double-blind trial. *N Engl J Med* 1974;291: 934–937.
9. Ehrenfeld M, Brzezinski A, Levy M, et al. Fertility and obstetric history in patients with familial Mediterranean fever on long-term colchicine therapy. *Br J Obstet Gynaecol* 1987;94:1186–1191.
10. Amoura Z, Schermann JM, Wechsler B, et al. Transplacental passage of colchicine in familial Mediterranean fever. *J Rheumatol* 1994;21:383.
11. Douglas GC, King BF. Colchicine inhibits human trophoblast differentiation in vitro. *Placenta* 1993;14:187–201.
12. Levy M, Yaffe C. Testicular function in patients with familial Mediterranean fever on long-term colchicine treatment. *Fertil Steril* 1978;29:667–668.
13. Haimov-Kochman R, Ben-Chetrit E. The effect of colchicine treatment on sperm production and function: a review. Hum Reprod 1998;13:360–362.
14. Sanders CL, Lucas MJ. Renal disease in pregnancy. *Obstet Gynecol Clin North Am* 2001;28:593–600.
15. Zemer D, Pras M, Sohar E, et al. Colchicine in the prevention and treatment of the amyloidosis of familial Mediterranean fever. *N Engl J Med* 1986;314:1001–1005.

16. Rubinow A, Cohen AS, Kayne H, et al. Colchicine therapy in amyloidosis. A preliminary report. *Arthritis Rheum* 1981;24(Suppl 1):S124.
17. Livneh A, Cabili S, Zemer D, et al. Effect of pregnancy on renal function in amyloidosis of familial Mediterranean fever. *J Rheumatol* 1993;20:1519–1523.
18. Zemer D, Livneh A, Pras M, et al. Familial Mediterranean fever in the colchicine era: the fate of one family. *Am J Med Genet* 1993;45: 340–344.
19. Shimoni Y, Shalev E. Pregnancy and complicated familial Mediterranean fever. *Int J Gynaecol Obstet* 1990;33:165–169.
20. Ditkoff EC, Sauer MV. Successful pregnancy in a familial Mediterranean fever patient following assisted reproduction. *J Assist Reprod Genet* 1996;13:684–685.
21. Zemer D, Pras M, Sohar E, et al. Colchicine in familial Mediterranean fever [letter]. *N Engl J Med* 1976;294:170–171.
22. Rabinovitch O, Zemer D, Kukia E, et al. Colchicine treatment in conception and pregnancy: two hundred thirty-one pregnancies in patients with familial Mediterranean fever. *Am J Reprod Immunol* 1992;28:245–246.

CHAPTER 15

USE OF WARFARIN DURING PREGNANCY

Adrienne Einarson, RN
Gideon Koren, MD, FRCPC

QUESTION

One of my patients, who has been taking warfarin for some time for treatment and prophylaxis of deep vein thrombosis, became pregnant due to failed contraception. I am unsure how to counsel her. Is there evidence that warfarin use during pregnancy is associated with fetal risk?

Answer

If possible, warfarin therapy should be avoided during pregnancy. If warfarin therapy is essential, it should be avoided at least during the first trimester (because of teratogenicity) and from about 2 to 4 weeks before delivery to reduce risk of hemorrhagic complications. Unfractionated heparin or low molecular weight heparin could be substituted when appropriate because these agents do not cross the placenta and are considered the anticoagulant drugs of choice during pregnancy.

Warfarin (Coumadin) is an oral anticoagulant that inhibits synthesis of vitamin K-dependent clotting factors, including factors II, VII, IX, and X, and the anticoagulant proteins C and S.[1] Rats given very high doses (100 mg/kg) of warfarin have had offspring with marked maxillonasal hypoplasia and skeletal abnormalities, including abnormal calcium bridges in the epiphysial cartilages of the vertebrae and long bones.[2]

STUDIES IN HUMAN BEINGS

Several case series and case reports of human use of warfarin during pregnancy have been published. These reports (which range in size from 1 to 418 subjects) show a clear association between warfarin therapy and embryopathy. The exact risk of fetal damage from warfarin therapy during pregnancy is difficult to determine because most of the available studies are small and anecdotal.

Several reports have indicated, however, that using warfarin between 6 and 12 weeks' gestation is associated with *fetal warfarin syndrome*, which is most commonly manifested by nasal hypoplasia, stippled epiphyses, limb deformities, and respiratory distress. Also, use of warfarin during the second and third trimesters has been associated sporadically with central nervous system abnormalities, including mental retardation, microcephaly, optic atrophy, and blindness.[3–6]

Other fetal abnormalities reported with maternal warfarin use include absent or nonfunctioning kidneys, anal dysplasia, deafness, seizures, Dandy-Walker syndrome, and focal cerebellar atrophy.[7–9] Use of warfarin throughout pregnancy has been associated with hemorrhagic complications, premature births, spontaneous abortions, stillbirths, and death.[4,5,10–15]

One study[8] reported on 418 cases of warfarin exposure from conception to 38 weeks after birth. About 16% of all pregnancies ended in spontaneous abortions or stillbirths, and another 15% resulted in babies with abnormalities at birth. The abnormalities included skeletal malformations (e.g., stippling of cervical vertebrae, sacrum, and femurs; kyphoscoliosis; and nasal hypoplasia) bilateral optic atrophy leading to blindness, deafness, focal cerebral atrophy, respiratory distress, and seizures. Doses of warfarin ranged from 2.5 to 12.5 mg/day.

Salazar and colleagues[11] reported on 128 babies exposed to warfarin therapy from 0 to 38 weeks' gestation. About 8% of the 38 live-born infants displayed teratogenic effects of warfarin at birth, including nasal hypoplasia, choanal stenosis, and stippled epiphyses. When compared with 68 pregnancies where women's warfarin therapy had been replaced with 1 g of acetylsalicylic acid and 400 mg of dipyridamole daily at the onset of pregnancy, it was clear that the rate of spontaneous abortions was significantly higher in the warfarin group (28% vs. 10%). The rate of neonatal deaths was also higher in the warfarin group (2.3% vs. 0). The rate of stillbirths was approximately 7% in both groups. Warfarin dose was adjusted for a target prothrombin time of 2 to 2.5 times control in most women.[11]

Ayhan et al.[12] reported on 64 pregnancies: 47 were exposed to warfarin, 11 were exposed to heparin, and 6 were not exposed to anticoagulation drugs. In 20 pregnancies warfarin was discontinued after 36 weeks' gestation. Fetal wastage occurred in 25 (53%) pregnancies exposed to warfarin, 4 (36%) exposed to heparin, and only 1 (17%) with no exposure to anticoagulation drugs. Two (4%) babies were born with warfarin-related malformations, manifested by a single kidney, digit deformities, and cleft lip and palate. There were 19 (40%) spontaneous abortions and 4 (9%) stillbirths with warfarin, but only 1 (9%) spontaneous abortion and no stillbirths with heparin. Warfarin doses were not reported in this study.

Vitali et al.[13] reported on 98 pregnancies exposed to warfarin since conception. Warfarin was replaced with heparin in 6 cases 3 weeks before delivery, was discontinued in 6 women before term, and was maintained in 13 women throughout the whole pregnancy. There were 37 spontaneous abortions (38%) and 13 voluntary terminations (13%). Of the 47 live births, 2 (4%) had warfarin-associated malformations at birth, manifested by occipital bone abnormalities, nasal hypoplasia, severe choanal stenosis, and cleft palate. One baby died from respiratory insufficiency 4 hours after delivery, and four (9%) babies were born with hemorrhagic complications secondary to warfarin therapy. Warfarin doses were not specified in this study.

Vitale et al.[15] reported on 58 exposures to warfarin throughout pregnancy until 38 weeks' gestation. Although 31 (53%) babies were reported normal at birth, 27 (47%) had fetal complications: 22 (38%) spontaneous abortions, 1 (1.7%) stillbirth, 2 (3%) warfarin embryopathies, 1 (1.7%) ventricular septal defect, and 1 (1.7%) growth retardation. Warfarin doses in this study were adjusted for a target international normalized ratio (INR) of 2.5 to 3.5. When stratified according to dose, 22 (81%) complications occurred after exposure to doses >5 mg/day. The study concluded there was a close association between warfarin dose and fetal complications.

Finally, another study looked at 114 exposures to warfarin during pregnancy.[16] While 50 women took warfarin throughout pregnancy, the remaining 64 women received subcutaneous heparin during the first trimester and warfarin during the second and third trimesters. All the women's warfarin therapy was replaced by heparin 2 to 4 weeks before labor. Spontaneous abortions occurred in 22% of cases exposed to either warfarin or heparin, and stillbirths occurred in 9% of cases exposed to warfarin and 11% of cases exposed to heparin. No embryopathies were reported among the live births.

CONCLUSION

The literature suggests a strong association between maternal warfarin use and fetal adverse effects. The most recent review[17] recommends that women receiving long-term oral anticoagulation have warfarin replaced with unfractionated or low molecular weight heparin when they become pregnant. There have, however, been case reports of unfractionated heparin being associated with adverse pregnancy outcomes, such as fetal loss and maternal thrombocytopenia, hemorrhage, and osteoporosis.[15] Needless to say, the women in these studies were often sick, and their complications could have been caused by underlying illness. A study of 108 women who received low molecular weight heparin for thromboprophylaxis[18] showed no increase above baseline for fetal deaths or malformations.

Women of childbearing age taking warfarin should be using effective birth control methods. Risks and benefits of treatment should be discussed with each woman who plans to become or is pregnant while taking this drug.

REFERENCES

1. Canadian Pharmacists Association. *Compendium of Pharmaceuticals and Specialties*. Ottawa, Ont: Canadian Pharmacists Association; 2001.
2. Howe AM, Webster WS. The warfarin embryopathy: a rat model showing maxillonasal hypoplasia and other skeletal disturbances. *Teratology* 1992;46:379–390.
3. Holzgreve W, Carey JC, Hall BD. Warfarin-induced fetal abnormalities. *Lancet* 1976;2:914–915.
4. Born D, Martinez EE, Almeida PA, et al. Pregnancy in patients with prosthetic heart valves: the effects of anticoagulation on mother, fetus, and neonate. *Am Heart J* 1992;124:413–417.
5. Sareli P, England MJ, Berk MR, et al. Maternal and fetal sequelae of anticoagulation during pregnancy in patients with mechanical heart valve prosthesis. *Am J Cardiol* 1989;63:1462–1465.
6. Pillans PI, Coetzee EJ. Anticoagulation during pregnancy. *S Afr Med J* 1986;69:469.
7. Hall BD. Warfarin embryopathy and urinary tract anomalies: possible new association. *Am J Med Genet* 1989;34:292–293.
8. Hall JG, Pauli RM, Wilson KM. Maternal and fetal sequelae of anticoagulation during pregnancy. *Am J Med* 1980;68:122–140.
9. Oakley C. Pregnancy in patients with prosthetic heart valves. *BMJ* 1983;286:1680–1682.

10. Chong MK, Harvey D, de Swiet M. Follow-up study of children whose mothers were treated with warfarin during pregnancy. *Br J Obstet Gynaecol* 1984;91:1070–1073.

11. Salazar E, Zajamas A, Gutierrez N, et al. The problem of cardiac valve prostheses, anticoagulants, and pregnancy. *Circulation* 1984;70(Suppl. 1): 169–177.

12. Ayhan A, Yapar EG, Yucek K, et al. Pregnancy and its complications after cardiac valve replacement. *Int J Gynaecol Obstet* 1991;35:117–122.

13. Vitali E, Donnatelli F, Quaini E, et al. Pregnancy in patients with mechanical prosthetic heart valves. *J Cardiovasc Surg* 1986;27:221–227.

14. Lee PK, Wang RY, Chow JS, et al. Combined use of warfarin and adjusted subcutaneous heparin during pregnancy in patients with an artificial heart valve. *J Am Coll Cardiol* 1986;8:221–224.

15. Vitale N, De Feo M, De Santo LS, et al. Dose-dependent fetal complications of warfarin in pregnant women with mechanical heart valves. *J Am Coll Cardiol* 1999;33:1637–1641.

16. Sharouni E, Oakley CM. Outcome of pregnancy in women with valve prostheses. *Br Heart J* 1994;71:196–201.

17. Ginsberg J, Greer I, Hirsh J. Use of antithrombotic agents during pregnancy. *Chest* 2001;119(Suppl. 1):122S–131S.

18. Schneider DM, von Tempelhoff GF, Heilmann L. Retrospective evaluation of the safety and efficacy of low molecular weight heparin as thromboprophylaxis during pregnancy. *Am J Obstet Gynecol* 1997;177:1567–1568.

CHAPTER 16

CAN WE USE ANXIOLYTICS DURING PREGNANCY WITHOUT ANXIETY?: IN MODERATION

Gideon Koren, MD, FRCPC

QUESTION

One of my patients suffers from anxiety and was using lorazepam to treat it. When she became pregnant, she stopped the medication immediately, but now she is worried about the potential effect on the baby because she was using the drug just after conception. Is this class of drugs safe during pregnancy? What should she do if she needs antianxiety treatment during the rest of her pregnancy?

Answer

Evidence to date from cohort studies did not identify a notable association between use of benzodiazepines (BZDs) and increased risk of major malformations, including oral cleft. In contrast, data from case-control studies show a slightly increased risk of oral cleft. Hence, level 2 ultrasonography is recommended to rule out visible forms of cleft lip. Using BZDs late in pregnancy could cause withdrawal syndrome in newborns.

BZDs are commonly used for anxiety and insomnia, even by pregnant women. A recent study found that 2% of pregnant women in the United States who were receiving Medicaid benefits filled one or more prescriptions for BZDs during pregnancy.[1] An international drug use study has shown that BZDs account for the greatest number (85%) of psychotropic agents used during pregnancy.[2] Because about half of pregnancies are unplanned,[3] many women could inadvertently expose fetuses to BZDs during the first trimester.

Antepartum exposure to BZDs has been associated with teratogenic effects (facial cleft, skeletal anomalies) in some animal studies[4,5] but not others.[6-7] Risk for cleft palate in the general population is approximately 0.06%.[8] Early human case-control studies suggested that maternal exposure to BZDs increases risk of fetal cleft lip and cleft palate.[9,10] Subsequent reports have implicated BZDs in other major malformations,[11-13] abnormal neurodevelopment,[11,14,15] and an irreproducible congenital benzodiazepine syndrome similar to fetal alcohol syndrome.[11,16-17]

Unfortunately, these studies were not designed to control for confounding factors that could influence results. Several prospective cohort studies involving hundreds of women using BZDs during pregnancy and an equal number of controls failed to show increased risk of malformations after BZD use during the first trimester.

The contradictory results mentioned above have led to considerable controversy surrounding use of BZDs during pregnancy.[18] Nevertheless, it seemed clear that, even if it existed, the risk of malformations in newborns exposed to BZDs during the first trimester was marginal. To investigate this issue, Motherisk conducted a meta-analysis of all data on exposure to BZDs during the first trimester.[19]

MOTHERISK'S META-ANALYSIS

Motherisk considered 13 studies that examined major malformations, 11 that examined oral cleft alone, and 3 that examined other specific malformations. Exposure was ascertained mainly through interviewing the mothers (61%), and outcome was confirmed mainly through examination by a physician, records (44%), or malformation registries (30%). Various BZDs were used or prescribed, although 48% of the studies examined use of chlorodiazepoxide or diazepam only.

Data pooled from seven cohort studies did not show an association between fetal exposure to BZDs during pregnancy and major malformations (Table 16-1). A combination of four case-control studies, however, showed that major malformations were associated with use of BZDs during pregnancy (Table 16-1). Data pooled from three cohort studies showed no association between fetal exposure to BZDs during pregnancy and oral cleft (Table 16-2), but analysis of six case-control studies produced a significant odds ratio for oral cleft.

TABLE 16-1
ASSOCIATION BETWEEN PRENATAL EXPOSURE TO BENZODIAZEPINES
AND MAJOR MALFORMATIONS

Studies	Malformed Exposed	Malformed Not Exposed	Odds Ratio (95% Confidence Interval)
Cohort			
Milkovich and van den Berg[13]	5/86	10/229	1.35 (0.45–4.07)
Crombie et al.[20]	3/300	382/19 143	0.75 (0.24–2.35)
Hartz et al.[21]	11/257	2129/46 233	0.90 (0.49–1.66)
Kullander and Kallen[22]	2/89	198/5664	0.63 (0.16–2.60)
Laegreid et al.[14]	1/17	1/29	1.75 (0.10–29.92)
Pastuszak et al.[23]	1/106	3/115	0.36 (0.04–3.47)
Ornoy et al.[24]	9/335	10/363	0.97 (0.39–2.43)
Combined effect			0.90 (0.61–1.35)
Case-Control			
Greenberg et al.[25]	36/60	800/1612	1.52 (0.9–2.58)
Bracken and Holford[26]	39/72	1331/4266	2.61 (1.63–4.16)
Noya[27]	1/24	0/24	3.13 (0.12–80.68)
Laegreid et al.[17]	8/10	10/68	23.20 (4.29–15.5)
Combined effect			3.01 (1.32–6.84)

DISCUSSION

Data from cohort studies showed no significant association between BZDs during the first trimester and either major malformations or oral cleft alone. Data from case-control studies, however, showed a small but significant increased risk for these outcomes. This finding might

TABLE 16-2
ASSOCIATION BETWEEN PRENATAL EXPOSURE TO BENZODIAZEPINES
AND ORAL CLEFT

Studies	Malformed Exposed	Malformed Not Exposed	Odds Ratio (95% Confidence Interval)
Cohort			
Shiono and Mills[28]	1/854	31/32 395	1.22 (0.17–8.89)
Bergman[1]	0/1354	62/102 985	1.21 (0.17–8.71)
Ornoy et al.[24]	0/335	0/363	1.08 (0.07–17.39)
Combined effect			1.19 (0.34–4.15)
Case-Control			
Safra and Oakley[12]	7/16	42/262	4.07 (1.44–11.54)
Saxen and Saxen[9]	27/40	511/1044	2.17 (1.11–4.24)
Rosenberg et al.[29]	13/67	590/3011	0.99 (0.54–1.82)
Rodriguez et al.[31]	8/61	442/7990	2.58 (1.22–5.45)
Czeizel[30]	48/91	1153/2311	1.12 (0.74–1.71)
Laegreid et al.[17]	2/10	4/68	4.00 (0.63–25.43)
Combined effect			1.79 (1.13–2.82)

reflect the substantially higher sensitivity of case-control studies for examining risk of specific malformations.

Tests of heterogeneity also showed that the cohort studies were homogeneous for both major malformations and oral cleft, whereas the case-control studies for oral cleft were heterogeneous, which decreases the reliability of the marginally significant results. Even when a "worst case scenario" is assumed, BZDs do not seem to be major human teratogens but, because some cases of cleft lip can be visualized by fetal ultrasound, level 2 ultrasonography should be used to rule out this malformation.

REFERENCES

1. Bergman U, Rosa FW, Baum C, et al. Effects of exposure to benzodiazepine during fetal life. *Lancet* 1992;340:694–696.
2. Marchetti F, Romero M, Bonati M, et al. Use of psychotropic drugs during pregnancy. *Eur J Clin Pharmacol* 1993;45:495–501.
3. Skrabanek P. Smoking and statistical overkill. *Lancet* 1992;340:1208–1209.
4. Miller RP, Becker BA. Teratogenicity of oral diazepam and diphenylhydantoin in mice. *Toxicol Appl Pharmacol* 1975;32:53–61.
5. Walker BE, Patterson A. Induction of cleft palate in mice by tranquillizers and barbiturates. *Teratology* 1974;10:159–163.
6. Beall JR. Study of the teratogenic potential of oral diazepam and SCH 12041. *Can Med Assoc J* 1972;106:1061.
7. Chesley S, Lumpkin M, Schatzki A, et al. Prenatal exposure to benzodiazepine. I. Prenatal exposure to lorazepam in mice alters open-field activity and GABA receptor function. *Neuropharmacology* 1991;30:53–58.
8. Heinonen OP, Sloane D, Shapiro S. *Birth Defects and Drugs in Pregnancy: Maternal Drug Exposure and Congenital Malformations.* Littleton, MA: Publishing Sciences Group; 1977.
9. Saxen I, Saxen L. Association between maternal intake of diazepam and oral clefts. *Lancet* 1975;2:498.
10. Saxen I, Lahti A. Cleft lip and palate in Finland: incidence, secular, seasonal, and geographical variations. *Teratology* 1974;9:217–224.
11. Laegreid L, Olegard R, Walstrom J, et al. Teratogenic effects of benzodiazepine use during pregnancy. *J Pediatr* 1989;114:126–131.
12. Safra MJ, Oakley GP. Association between cleft lip with or without cleft palate and prenatal exposure to diazepam. *Lancet* 1975;2:478–480.
13. Milkovich L, van den Berg BJ. Effects of prenatal meprobamate and chlordiazepoxide hydrochloride on human embryonic and fetal development. *N Engl J Med* 1974;291:1268–1271.
14. Laegreid L, Hagberg G, Lundberg A. Neurodevelopment in late infancy after prenatal exposure to benzodiazepines a prospective study. *Neuropediatrics* 1992;23:60–67.
15. Viggedal G, Hagberg BS, Laegreid L, et al. Mental development in late infancy after prenatal exposure to benzodiazepines a prospective study. *J Child Psychol Psychiatry* 1993;34:295–305.
16. Laegreid L, Olegard R, Wahlstrom J, et al. Abnormalities in children exposed to benzodiazepines in utero. *Lancet* 1987;1:108–109.
17. Laegreid L, Olegard R, Conradi N, et al. Congenital malformations and maternal consumption of benzodiazepines: a case-control study. *Dev Med Child Neurol* 1990;32:432–441.
18. Dolovich L, Addis A, Vaillancourt JMR, et al. Benzodiazepine use in pregnancy and major malformations or oral cleft: meta-analysis of cohort and case-control studies *BMJ* 1998;317:839–843.
19. Winship KA, Cahal DA, Weber JP, et al. Maternal drug histories and central nervous system anomalies. *Arch Dis Child* 1984;59:1052–1060.
20. Crombie DL, Pinsent RJ, Fleming DM, et al. Fetal effects of tranquilizers in pregnancy. *N Engl J Med* 1975;293:198–199.

21. Hartz SC, Heinonen OP, Shapiro S, et al. Antenatal exposure to meprobamate and chlordiazepoxide in relation to malformations, mental development, and childhood mortality. *N Engl J Med* 1975;292:726–728.

22. Kullander S, Kallen B. A prospective study of drugs and pregnancy. I. Psychopharmaca. *Acta Obstet Gynecol Scand* 1976;55:25–33.

23. Pastuszak A, Milich V, Chan S, et al. Prospective assessment of pregnancy outcome following first trimester exposure to benzodiazepines. *Can J Clin Pharmacol* 1996;3:167–171.

24. Ornoy A, Moerman L, Lukashova I, et al. The outcome of children exposed in utero to benzodiazepines. *Teratology* 1997;55:102A.

25. Greenberg G, Inman WH, Weatherall JA, et al. Maternal drug histories and congenital abnormalities. *BMJ* 1977;2:853–856.

26. Bracken MB, Holford TR. Exposure to prescribed drugs in pregnancy and association with congenital malformations. *Obstet Gynecol* 1981;58:336–344.

27. Noya CA. Epidemiological study on congenital malformations. *Rev Cubana Hig Epidemiol* 1981;19:200–210.

28. Shiono PH, Mills JL. Oral clefts and diazepam use during pregnancy. *N Engl J Med* 1984;311:919–920.

29. Rosenberg L, Mitchell AA, Parsells JL, et al. Lack of relation of oral clefts to diazepam use during pregnancy. *N Engl J Med* 1983;309:1282–1285.

30. Czeizel A. Lack of evidence of teratogenicity of benzodiazepine drugs in Hungary. *Reprod Toxicol* 1987-88;1:183–188.

31. Rodriguez PE, Salvador PJ, Garcia AF, et al. Relationship between benzodiazepine ingestion during pregnancy and oral clefts in the newborn: a case-control study. *Med Clin* 1986;87:741–743.

CHAPTER 17

NAUSEA AND VOMITING OF PREGNANCY: EVIDENCE-BASED TREATMENT ALGORITHM

Caroline Maltepe, BA
Adrienne Einarson, RN
Gideon Koren, MD, FRCPC

QUESTION

One of my patients suffers from a moderate-to-severe form of morning sickness. She responded only partially to doxylamine and pyridoxine (Diclectin), and I wish to try adding another medication. What should my priority be?

Answer

An algorithm used by Motherisk to manage thousands of patients takes a hierarchical approach to this condition. This approach is evidence based with regard to fetal safety as well as efficacy.

Nausea and vomiting of pregnancy (NVP) affects an estimated 80% of all pregnant women, making it the most common medical condition during pregnancy.[1] In most cases, symptoms are worse in the morning; severity usually peaks by 8 to 12 weeks' gestation.[2] Some women are affected throughout the day, and the condition sometimes continues beyond the first trimester and even until the birth.[2]

Hyperemesis gravidarum is the most severe form of morning sickness, affecting 0.05% to 1% of pregnant women. Hyperemesis gravidarum is characterized by dehydration and electrolyte imbalance, and might require hospitalization. Nausea and vomiting of pregnancy has serious detrimental effects on the lives of women, even those with a milder presentation.[3] Termination of otherwise wanted pregnancies among women suffering from severe and prolonged NVP has been reported.[4]

INAPPROPRIATE TREATMENT COMMON

Ample evidence indicates that most women with NVP do not receive appropriate pharmacologic or nonpharmacologic treatment for the condition.[5] In 1996, the Motherisk Program in Toronto, Ont., initiated the NVP Healthline (1-800-436-8477) to counsel and support women and health professionals in managing NVP. Members of Motherisk systematically review available data on treatment in an attempt to obtain the best available evidence on efficacy and safety. Callers and clinic patients are advised on both pharmacologic and nonpharmacologic management.

This paper provides clinicians with a simple evidence-based algorithm on the efficacy and safety of treatments for NVP.

RATIONALE

In planning and evaluating management of NVP, fetal safety is clearly the primary concern, followed by efficacy. This order of priorities dictates that, in general, older medications, for which there are more data on fetal safety, are preferred over newer, perhaps more effective, drugs for which there are as yet fewer data on safety.

METHODS

The algorithm is based on a recent systematic review of the literature on safety and efficacy of management of NVP conducted by members of the Motherisk Team.[6] The course of NVP ranges in severity, length, and response to treatment. We addressed treatment of NVP in a decision tree (Fig. 17-1). It begins with pharmacologic management of relatively mild cases and progresses to treatment of patients who cannot tolerate oral treatment or are dehydrated, or both. At any stage of the algorithm, physicians can add or, when there is improvement, withdraw treatment. The systematic review[6] included meta-analyses whenever the data permitted.

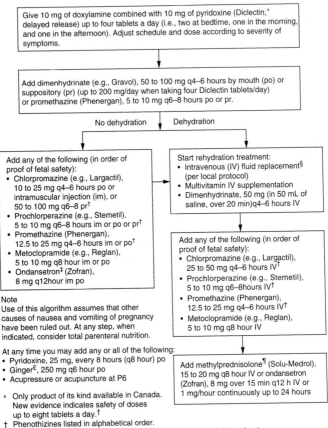

Give 10 mg of doxylamine combined with 10 mg of pyridoxine (Diclectin,* delayed release) up to four tablets a day (i.e., two at bedtime, one in the morning, and one in the afternoon). Adjust schedule and dose according to severity of symptoms.

Add dimenhydrinate (e.g., Gravol), 50 to 100 mg q4–6 hours by mouth (po) or suppository (pr) (up to 200 mg/day when taking four Diclectin tablets/day) or promethazine (Phenergan), 5 to 10 mg q6–8 hours po or pr.

No dehydration   Dehydration

Add any of the following (in order of proof of fetal safety):
- Chlorpromazine (e.g., Largactil), 10 to 25 mg q4–6 hours po or intramuscular injection (im), or 50 to 100 mg pr†
- Prochlorperazine (e.g., Stemetil), 5 to 10 mg q6–8 hours im or po or pr†
- Promethazine (Phenergan), 12.5 to 25 mg q4–6 hours im or po†
- Metoclopramide (e.g., Reglan), 5 to 10 mg q8 hour im or po
- Ondansetron‡ (Zofran), 8 mg q12hour im po

Start rehydration treatment:
- Intravenous (IV) fluid replacement§ (per local protocol)
- Multivitamin IV supplementation
- Dimenhydrinate, 50 mg (in 50 mL of saline, over 20 min)q4–6 hours IV

Add any of the following (in order of proof of fetal safety):
- Chlorpromazine (e.g., Largactil), 25 to 50 mg q4–6 hours IV†
- Prochlorperazine (e.g., Stemetil), 5 to 10 mg q6–8hours IV†
- Promethazine (Phenergan), 12.5 to 25 mg q4–6 hours IV†
- Metoclopramide (e.g., Reglan), 5 to 10 mg q8 hour IV

Note
Use of this algorithm assumes that other causes of nausea and vomiting of pregnancy have been ruled out. At any step, when indicated, consider total parenteral nutrition.

At any time you may add any or all of the following:
- Pyridoxine, 25 mg, every 8 hours (q8 hour) po
- Ginger£, 250 mg q6 hour po
- Acupressure or acupuncture at P6

Add methylprednisolone¶ (Solu-Medrol), 15 to 20 mg q8 hour IV or ondansetron (Zofran), 8 mg over 15 min q12 h IV or 1 mg/hour continuously up to 24 hours

* Only product of its kind available in Canada. New evidence indicates safety of doses up to eight tablets a day.†
† Phenothizines listed in alphabetical order.
‡ Safety perticularly during first trimester of pregnancy, not yet determined.
§ No study line compared various fluid replacements for nausa and vemating during pregnancy.
£ Safety of dose >1000 mg/day not yet determined for pregnancy.
¶ Steroids not recomended during first 10 weeks of pregnancy because of possible increased risk of oral clafte.

F I G U R E   1 7 - 1   *Decision tree*

The quality of the evidence on fetal safety and maternal efficacy varies. There is large and convincing evidence on the safety and efficacy of doxylamine and pyridoxine (Diclectin). Evidence on the safety of other H_1 blockers is as strong, but evidence of efficacy is less strong. Many studies on the efficacy of phenothiazines offer convincing evidence, but the number of studies on safety is much smaller (birth defects are generally rare). Evidence on the safety and efficacy of ondansetron and metoclopramide is preliminary. New studies fail to show teratogenicity of ginger, metoclopamide, and andansetron.

The hierarchy presented in the algorithm is based on the strength of evidence for fetal safety, and only treatments shown to be efficacious were included. It has been used by the Motherisk Program for treating a large number of patients.

REFERENCES

1. Gadsby R, Barnie-Adshead AM, Jagger C. A prospective study of nausea and vomiting during pregnancy. *Br J Gen Pract* 1993;43:245–248.
2. O'Brien B, Zhou Q. Variables related to nausea and vomiting during pregnancy. *Birth* 1995;22:93–100.
3. Mazzotta P, Stewart D, Atanackovic G, et al. Psychosocial morbidity among women with nausea and vomiting of pregnancy: prevalence and association with anti-emetic therapy. *J Psychosom Obstet Gynaecol* 2000;21:129–136.
4. Mazzota P, Magee L, Koren G. Therapeutic abortions due to severe morning sickness. Unacceptable combination. *Can Fam Physician* 1997;43:1055–1057.
5. Mazzotta P, Maltepe C, Navioz Y, et al. Attitudes, management and consequences of nausea and vomiting of pregnancy in the United States and Canada. *Int J Gynaecol Obstet* 2000;70:359–365.
6. Mazzotta P, Magee LA. A risk-benefit assessment of pharmacological and nonpharmacological treatment of nausea and vomiting of pregnancy. *Drugs* 2000;59(4):781–800.
7. Atanackovic G, Navioz Y, Moretti ME, et al. The safety of higher than standard dose of doxylamine-pyridoxine (Diclectin) for nausea and vomiting of pregnancy. *J Clin Pharmacol* 2001;41:842–845.

CAN HERBAL PRODUCTS BE USED SAFELY DURING PREGNANCY?

Gideon Koren, MD, FRCPC

QUESTION

Many of my patients are now using herbal medicines; some even use them during pregnancy. As we enter the "cold and flu" season, many are inquiring about use of the herb echinacea to prevent these ailments. Is there any evidence to suggest that use of echinacea during pregnancy is safe?

Answer

Although herbal products have been used in the past during pregnancy and delivery, there is little evidence showing they are safe. Many authoritative reviews of echinacea report that its safety for use during pregnancy has not been established. A recent Motherisk study showed that use of echinacea during the first trimester of pregnancy was not associated with increased risk of major malformations.

Use of herbal medicine, or phytomedicine, has increased in popularity. Statistics Canada reported that at least 3.3 million Canadians spent more than $1 billion in 1995 on some form of complementary or alternative medicine not covered by a health plan.[1] In particular, women have been documented as frequent users of complementary or alternative therapies.[2,3] In 1996, nearly 60% of Canadian women believed that herbal remedies were helpful in preventing and treating illness.[4] These herbal products are often used during pregnancy with the assumption that "natural" is synonymous with "safe."

In two separate studies, more than 50% of general practitioners in Canada were shown to have referred their patients for complementary or alternative therapies.[5,6] A Motherisk study showed that 98% of surveyed physicians reported that their patients routinely discussed complementary or alternative medicine with them even though 74% of the physicians were unsure about the safety of herbal products during pregnancy.[7] Although MEDLINE citations on "alternative medicine" are growing at twice the annual rate of the overall medical literature,[8] few of these articles describe controlled studies, and even fewer address the safety of these medicinals during pregnancy. Health-care providers are normally left with the difficult task of evaluating the safety and risk of herbs without benefit of clinical or evidence-based information.

The popularity of these products and the limited information available has meant that the Motherisk Program has experienced an increased number of women and health care providers inquiring about the safety and risks of herbal remedies during pregnancy. To address these concerns, Motherisk has systematically reviewed the available literature and formed a database of frequently discussed herbs. The most common of these appear in *Maternal—Fetal Toxicology: A Clinician's Guide*, 3rd edition.[9] Herbs are identified by species and family names, and their primary constituents and pharmacologic actions discussed. At standardized doses, adverse effects, cautions, contraindications, and drug interactions are outlined. Reported clinical cases and theoretical concerns are noted (Table 18-1[9]).

Two of the most common herbal preparations discussed over the counseling line and by patients in general are echinacea and St John's wort.[5] The Motherisk Program is currently conducting a prospective controlled study on St John's wort during pregnancy and following up mothers who use the herb during lactation.

The first prospective controlled study addressing the safety of herbs during pregnancy was completed using the herb echinacea.[10] A total of 206 women who used echinacea products during pregnancy were enrolled into the study (112 used it during the first trimester). This cohort was disease-matched (upper respiratory tract ailments) to women exposed to nonteratogenic agents by maternal age and alcohol and cigarette use. Results of this study suggest that use of echinacea during organogenesis is not associated with increased risk for major malformations.

As use of herbal medicine continues to grow, patients will call upon their physicians to answer questions about the safety of these products. Aside from our recent study on use of echinacea, no other studies addressing safety during pregnancy have been completed.

TABLE 18-1.

Echinacea: *E angustifolia DC, E purpurea (L) Moench, E pallida (Nutt) Nutt, Asteraceae*
Primary constituents: carbohydrates (polysaccharides), glycoproteins, amides (alkamides); caffeic acid derivatives (echinacoside, cichoric acid, cynarin). Although the three species are often considered interchangeable, their chemical constituents do differ.
Primary pharmacologic actions: Immunostimulatory, anti-inflammatory, antibacterial, antiviral, antineoplastic
Common uses: Upper respiratory tract (common cold and flu) and lower respiratory tract infections
Dose • Dried herb: 1 g three times daily • Liquid extract: 0.25 to 1.0 mL three times daily • Tincture: 1 to 2 mL three times daily
Adverse effects/toxicology: No reported toxicity
Cautions/contraindications: Should be avoided by people with known allergy to sunflower *(Asteraceae)* family. Use with caution for patients with progressive systemic diseases (tuberculosis, multiple sclerosis) and autoimmune conditions (diabetes mellitus, lupus, rheumatoid arthritis)
Drug interactions: Immunostimulatory action suggests caution with immunosuppressant agents
Implications for pregnancy and lactation: A prospective controlled study completed by the Motherisk Program and analysis of first-trimester cases (N = 112) suggests that the difference in the rate of major malformations between the study group and the disease-matched control group is not statistically significant. Safety during lactation has not been established

Adapted with permission from Gallo et al.[9]

Women and their health care providers should discuss openly the potential for reproductive or adverse effects when herbs are used during pregnancy.

REFERENCES

1. Immen W. Clinic to open doors to alternative medicine. *Globe and Mail* 1996 July 1;Sect. A:1.
2. Beal M. Women's use of complementary and alternative therapies in reproductive health care. *J Nurse Midwifery* 1998;43(3):224–234.

3. MacLennan A, Wilson D, Taylor A. Prevalence and cost of alternative medicine in Australia. *Lancet* 1996;347:569–573.
4. Angus Reid Group. 1996 family health study. *Can Living* 1996;11:157.
5. Verhoef MJ, Sutherland LR. Alternative medicine and general practitioners: opinions and behaviour. *Can Fam Physician* 1995;41:1005–1011.
6. LaValley JW, Verhoef MJ. Integrating complementary medicine and health care services into practice. *Can Med Assoc J* 1995;153:45–49.
7. Einarson A, Lawrimore T, Brand P, et al. Attitudes and practices of physicians and naturopaths toward herbal products, including use during pregnancy and lactation. *Can J Clin Pharmacol* 2000; 7(1):45–49.
8. Petrie K, Peck M. Alternative medicine in maternity care. *Prim Care* 2000;27(1):117–136.
9. Gallo M, Smith M, Boon H, et al. The use of herbal medicine in pregnancy and lactation: a clinician's guide. In: Koren G. Maternal-fetal toxicology. New York, NY: Marcel Dekker; 2001. p. 569–602.
10. Gallo M, Sarkar M, Au W, et al. Pregnancy outcome following gestational exposure to echinacea: a prospective controlled study. *Arch Intern Med* 2000;160:3141–3143.

CHAPTER 19

TAKING ACE INHIBITORS DURING PREGNANCY: IS IT SAFE?

Gideon Koren, MD, FRCPC

QUESTION

A pregnant patient is taking enalapril for primary hypertension. How safe are angiotensin-converting enzyme inhibitors (ACEI) during pregnancy?

Answer

Evidence of whether ACEIs cause problems during the first trimester of pregnancy is reassuring. There is evidence that they cause severe renal and other problems during the second and third trimesters, however. These drugs should be avoided during pregnancy.

Incidence of chronic hypertension during pregnancy ranges from 0.5% to 3.0% depending on the population studied.[1] Maternal and perinatal morbidity and mortality are generally not increased when patients have uncomplicated mild chronic hypertension. Risks to both mother and fetus increase dramatically, however, when pregnancy is complicated by severe uncontrolled hypertension or other risk factors, such as older maternal age, hypertension lasting more than 15 years, diabetes, renal disease, cardiac disease, or connective tissue disease.[1] Some reported complications of uncontrolled hypertension during pregnancy are maternal death, stroke, heart failure, and pulmonary edema; common fetal complications are intrauterine growth restriction, abruption of the placenta, and prematurity and its adverse effects.[1]

ACEI are excellent antihypertensive agents with few side effects (Table 19-1). They are becoming widely used as first-line therapy for chronic hypertension in women of reproductive age. They are also

TABLE 19-1.
ANGIOTENSIN-CONVERTING ENZYME INHIBITORS

Agent	Trade Name	Agent	Trade Name
Benazepril	Lotensin	Captopril	Capoten
Cilazapril	Inhibace	Enalapril	Vasotec
Enalaprilat	Vasotec IV	Fosinopril	Monopril
Lisinopril	Prinivil, Zestril	Perindopril	Coversyl
Quinapril	Acupril	Ramipril	Altace

used in treatment of renovascular hypertension, autoimmune diseases, and diabetes mellitus in this age group. Because 50% of all pregnancies are unplanned, some women are bound to be taking ACEIs at the time of conception.

ANIMAL STUDIES

Animal studies of rats and rabbits given ACEIs during organogenesis showed no increased incidence of major malformations in offspring. Animal data reveal, however, increased morbidity and mortality in fetuses exposed to ACEIs in utero. Decreased uteroplacental blood flow, low birth weight, hypotension, preterm delivery, and fetal death were noted.[2] A prospective placebo-controlled study of baboons showed a significant increase in fetal death or fetal growth restriction (4 of 13) in the group treated with enalapril compared with no instances among the controls.[3]

PLACENTAL TRANSFER

Captopril, enalapril, and lisinopril have been shown to cross the human placenta in pharmacologically significant amounts; other ACEIs probably do the same.[4-6] Once in a fetus, most ACEIs are excreted renally in their active form (when there is urine production) and could be recirculated through swallowed amniotic fluid.

FIRST-TRIMESTER EXPOSURE

Postmarketing surveillance of ACEI use during the first trimester of pregnancy in the United States, Canada, and Israel followed the outcomes of 79 women who had been exposed to ACEIs. Among the 66 women exposed during only the first trimester (<14 weeks), there were 48 live births (including 2 sets of twins), 15 spontaneous abortions, and 5 therapeutic abortions. Among the 48 live births, 3 cases of intrauterine growth restriction were documented. One case involved twins delivered at 36 weeks' gestation; the other two cases involved full-term infants. Another child had a patent ductus arteriosus that required surgical ligation at 18 months. This infant was born at 40 weeks' gestation to a mother who discontinued ACEI treatment at 7 weeks' gestation and was treated with digoxin throughout the pregnancy and warfarin sodium for the first 5 weeks followed by heparin for the remainder of the pregnancy. No babies who had been exposed to ACEIs during only the first trimester had renal tubular dysplasia. Among the 13 mothers who continued ACEI treatment beyond 14 weeks' gestation, there were 13 live births with 1 major malformation (renal tubular dysplasia).[7]

A surveillance study of Michigan Medicaid recipients involved 86 newborns exposed to captopril during the first trimester. Four newborns (4.7%) had major birth defects, including one cardiovascular anomaly, one polydactyly, one limb reduction defect, and one hypospadias. In a review by Briggs et al.,[8] among 40 newborns exposed to enalapril during the first trimester, 4 (10%) had major birth defects, including 2 cardiovascular anomalies and 1 polydactyly, and among 15 newborns exposed to lisinopril during the first trimester, 2 (13.3%) had major birth defects, including 1 polydactyly.

A European survey[9] reviewed pregnancy outcome of 22 women treated with captopril and 9 women treated with enalapril; 21 women conceived while they were taking ACEIs and 15 continued therapy until the end of pregnancy. Most women (27 of 31) had chronic essential hypertension, and 3 were proteinuric before pregnancy. No malformations were reported among the 14 pregnancies exposed to captopril during the first trimester. In the enalapril group, there were two spontaneous abortions in two women exposed during the first trimester, one at 7 weeks and the other at 11 weeks, both attributed to other causes. In a third case where enalapril was started at 24 weeks for severe glomerulopathy, a stillborn infant was delivered after 2 weeks. In six cases where women were taking enalapril at the time of conception, four discontinued treatment at 7 weeks, one discontinued at 28 weeks, and one continued throughout pregnancy (40 weeks): two infants were small for dates (one exposed throughout pregnancy, the other during only the first trimester). No other anomalies were mentioned.

SECOND- AND THIRD-TRIMESTER EXPOSURE

In contrast to first-trimester exposure to ACEIs, second- and third-trimester exposure appears to be fetotoxic, producing fetal hypocalvaria and renal defects. The cause of these defects appears to be related to fetal hypotension and reduced renal blood flow. Anuria associated with oligohydramnios can produce fetal limb contractures, craniofacial deformations, and pulmonary hypoplasia. Intrauterine growth restriction, prematurity, persistence of patent ductus arteriosus, severe neonatal hypotension, neonatal anuria, and neonatal or fetal death have all been observed with use of these drugs.[10]

Infants affected by use of ACEIs during pregnancy have been born to mothers with hypertension of varying etiology. Although maternal hypertension might produce oligohydramnios, fetal growth restriction, and fetal distress, the evolution of oligohydramnios followed by delivery of a hypotensive anuric infant has not been described as one of the complications of maternal hypertension and is probably drug induced. There are case reports of resolution of oligohydramnios after discontinuation of ACEIs, and angiotensin-converting enzyme activity in exposed neonates was found to be profoundly blunted and normalized only after the renally excreted drug was removed by dialysis.[10-12]

There are several cases of oligohydramnios, fetal hypocalvaria, fetal renal damage, and fetal death reported in association with use of ACEIs during the second and third trimesters of pregnancy.[8-12] Twenty-nine cases of perinatal renal failure in association with maternal use of ACEIs were listed by the United States Federal Drug Administration in 1991.[13]

In a 1991 summary of 85 pregnancies during which women were exposed to ACEIs, 11 deaths (perinatal mortality rate 13%), including 6 stillbirths and 5 neonatal deaths, were reported.[14] Based on limited epidemiologic data, the morbidity from exposure to ACEIs in the second and third trimesters of pregnancy is estimated to be as high as 10% to 20%. Another article published in 1998 reporting pregnancy outcome in 20 prospective cases and reviewing 85 published cases stated that reported anomaly rates were lower in a larger series.[15]

Some women with severe uncontrolled hypertension might have to take ACEIs during pregnancy.[16] In a small series of 10 patients with severe unresponsive hypertension, low-dose captopril was shown to improve maternal well-being with no fetal or neonatal compromise.[17] The small sample size, however, might not have been able to detect a 5% to 10% risk of fetal morbidity or mortality. Case reports of use of angiotensin-2 receptor inhibitors during pregnancy show fetal effects similar to those observed with ACEIs.[18]

CONCLUSION

It is advisable not to prescribe ACEIs for pregnant women. Although there is insufficient evidence to ensure that ACEIs are safe if taken during the first trimester, they do not appear to be major teratogens. If women have to be treated with ACEIs during the second or third trimesters of pregnancy, close monitoring with serial sonograms for assessing amniotic fluid volume and fetal growth are necessary. Although oligohydramnios has been observed to reverse once ACEIs are discontinued, it should be remembered that oligohydramnios often does not appear until after a fetus has sustained irreversible injury. Renal function and blood pressure should be closely monitored in newborns exposed to ACEIs in utero.

REFERENCES

1. James DK, Steer PJ, Weiner CP, et al. *High-risk pregnancy management options.* London, England: Saunders Company Ltd; 1996.
2. Mastrobattista JM. Angiotensin-converting enzyme inhibitors in pregnancy. *Semin Perinatol* 1997;21:124–134.
3. Harewood WJ, Phippard AF, Duggin GG, et al. Fetotoxicity of angiotensin-converting enzyme inhibition in primate pregnancy: a prospective, placebo-controlled study in baboons *(Papio hamadryas). Am J Obstet Gynecol* 1994;171:633–642.
4. Reisenberger K, Egarter C, Sternberger B, et al. Placental passage of angiotensin-converting enzyme inhibitors. *Am J Obstet Gynecol* 1996;174:1450–1455.
5. Schubiger G, Flury G, Nusserberger J. Enalapril for pregnancy-induced hypertension: acute renal failure in a neonate. *Ann Intern Med* 1988; 108:215–216.
6. Pyrde PG, Sedman AB, Nugent CE, et al. Angiotensin-converting enzyme inhibitor fetopathy. *J Am Soc Nephrol* 1993;3:1575–1582.
7. Centers for Disease Control and Prevention. Post marketing surveillance for angiotensin-converting enzyme inhibitor use during the first trimester

of pregnancy United States, Canada, and Israel, 1987–1995. *JAMA* 1997;277(5):1193–1194.

8. Briggs GG, Freeman RK, Yaffe SJ. Drugs in pregnancy and lactation. Baltimore, Md: Williams & Wilkins; 1998.

9. Kreft-Jais C, Plouin PF, Tchobroutsky C, et al. Angiotensin-converting enzyme inhibitors in pregnancy: a survey of 22 patients given captopril and nine given enalapril. *Br J Obstet Gynaecol* 1988;95(4):420–422.

10. Barr M Jr. Teratogen update: angiotensin-converting enzyme inhibitors. *Teratology* 1994;50:399–409.

11. ACE inhibitors in pregnancy [letters]. *Lancet* 1989;2:96–97.

12. Cunniff C, Jones KL, Phillipson J, et al. Oligohydramnios sequence and renal tubular malformation associated with maternal enalapril use. *Am J Obstet Gynecol* 1990;162:187–189.

13. Rosa F, Bosco L, Graham CF, et al. Neonatal anuria with maternal angiotensin-converting enzyme inhibition. *Obstet Gynecol* 1989;74:371–374.

14. Hanssens M, Keirse MJ, Vankelecom F, et al. Fetal and neonatal effects of treatment with angiotensin-converting enzyme inhibitors in pregnancy. *Obstet Gynecol* 1991;78:128–135.

15. Burrows RF, Burrows EA. Assessing the teratogenic potential of angiotensin-converting enzyme inhibitors in pregnancy. *Aust N Z J Obstet Gynaecol* 1998;38(3):306–311.

16. Pryde PG, Barr M Jr. Low-dose, short-acting, angiotensin-converting enzyme inhibitors as rescue therapy in pregnancy [letter]. *Obstet Gynecol* 2001;97(5 Pt 1):799–800.

17. Easterling TR, Carr DB, Davis C, et al. Low-dose, short-acting, angiotensin-converting enzyme inhibitors as rescue therapy in pregnancy. *Obstet Gynecol* 2000;96(6):956–961.

18. Chung NA, Lip GY, Beevers M, et al. Angiotensin-II-receptor inhibitors in pregnancy. *Lancet* 2001;357(9268):1620–1621.

CHAPTER 20

PROLONGED EXPOSURE TO ANGIOTENSIN-CONVERTING ENZYME INHIBITORS DURING PREGNANCY. FETAL TOXICITY COULD BE REVERSIBLE

Alon Shrim, MD
Gideon Koren, MD, FRCPC

QUESTION

I read in a Motherisk update that angiotensin-converting enzyme (ACE) inhibitors are contraindicated during pregnancy. Many women, however, do not know they are pregnant for quite some time after conception. One of my patients was taking ACE inhibitors for 3 to 4 months while she was pregnant. How should I advise her?

Answer

The deleterious effects ACE inhibitors have on fetuses were seen only after exposure during the second and third trimesters and were mostly secondary to renal damage. These effects can be reversed, as described in this Motherisk update.

ACE inhibitors are first-line medications in treatment of hypertension and cardiac and renal diseases. Investigators consistently report fetal toxicity after maternal exposure to ACE inhibitors during late pregnancy. Adverse effects include fetal renal dysplasia, oligohydramnios, intrauterine growth restriction, skull hypoplasia, patent ductus arteriosus, pulmonary hypoplasia, and deformities of the limbs.[1] Approximately half of all pregnancies are unplanned,[2] so physicians should be prepared to give accurate information and counseling to women who take ACE inhibitors during pregnancy. We thought it would be useful to present a case where there were sonographic signs of fetal ACE-inhibitor toxicity and then a favorable outcome after the ACE inhibitor was discontinued.

CASE

A 28-year-old woman in her second pregnancy was referred to Mount Sinai Hospital in Toronto, Ont, for evaluation at 25.5 weeks' gestation. Her medical history included chronic renal disease and hypertension secondary to mixed connective tissue disease. She was taking 60 mg of nifedipine, 50 mg of atenolol, 200 mg of hydroxychloroquine, and 50 mg of ramipril (an ACE inhibitor) each day.

Her current pregnancy had been diagnosed only 3 weeks before the referral. At that time, she had had an ultrasound scan that demonstrated fetal biometry consistent with a fetus of 22 weeks' gestation. Fetal anatomy was normal, but severe oligohydramnios was noted. Otherwise, the pregnancy appeared to be uncomplicated. Following the scan, the ramipril was discontinued, and her dosage of atenolol was increased.

Three weeks later, a detailed ultrasound examination revealed that the amniotic fluid volume had returned to normal with an index of 15.3. Fetal anatomy was normal, except for the presence of a two-vessel cord. Appropriate fetal body and breathing movements were seen. Results of Doppler scans of the umbilical artery and the middle cerebral artery were normal. Estimated fetal weight was at the 15th percentile for 25 weeks' gestation. No further deterioration in the fetus' condition was noted, but at 30 weeks' gestation, the patient was admitted for cesarean section because of worsening hypertension and renal function.

An 880-g female infant was delivered, with Apgar scores of 8 and 9 at 1 and 5 minutes of age, respectively. Because of increasing respiratory distress, she was intubated at 90 minutes of age and received two doses of surfactant. She was ventilated for 6 days, and she needed continuous positive airway pressure for 14 days. She developed mild physiologic jaundice with a maximum bilirubin level of 197 mmol/L on day 8. Results of an ultrasound scan of her head were normal. She was passing 4 to 6 mL/kg of urine hourly from day 1. Her renal function tests showed abnormally high initial levels that eventually settled in the first 48 hours. Her creatinine levels were 188, 148, 112, 72, and 58 mmol/L and her urea level was 12.2, 17.4, 15.6, 7.3, and 5.8 mmol/L at 24, 36, 48, 60, and 120 hours old, respectively.

MECHANISM

Studies in animals have shown a high incidence of fetal death and still-birth with use of ACE inhibitors during pregnancy.[3,4] The deleterious fetal outcomes, namely oligohydramnios, intrauterine growth restriction, skull hypoplasia, patent ductus arteriosus, oligohydramnios-related pulmonary hypoplasia, and limb deformities, result from two mechanisms: damage to fetal kidneys and a decrease in uterine blood flow that leads to decreased oxygen delivery to the fetus.[5] These conditions are secondary to the direct effect of an ACE inhibitor on the fetal renin-angiotensin system.[6,7]

EPIDEMIOLOGY

Epidemiologic evidence regarding fetal ACE-inhibitor toxicity is based mostly on case reports and case studies. It is important to note that no teratogenic effects were noted in reports of infants exposed to ACE inhibitors (mainly captopril or enalapril) during only the first trimester.[8–10] In contrast, there is concern when use of ACE inhibitors continues into the second and third trimesters. This concern is increasing as reports of grave fetal outcomes are being published frequently.[11]

The exact rate of severe adverse fetal or neonatal outcomes can only be estimated in the absence of cohort studies. One obstacle in estimating the effect of ACE inhibitors on a fetus is the confounding effect of maternal disease. As in the case presented here, hypertension treated with ACE inhibitors might have various causes, including some very severe maternal conditions, such as lupus erythematosus and renal transplantation. These underlying conditions themselves could contribute to adverse fetal outcomes. Although data are limited, there does not appear to be a strong teratogenic risk for women exposed to ACE inhibitors when they conceive.[12]

Discontinuation of ACE inhibitors before the second trimester is recommended by the U.S. Food and Drug Administration because of the effects seen in both humans and animals. As our case demonstrates, however, poor neonatal outcome after prolonged exposure to ACE inhibitors is not inevitable, and the effect of long-term antenatal exposure to ACE inhibitors could be reversible.

REFERENCES

1. Mastrobattista JM. Angiotensin-converting enzyme inhibitors in pregnancy. *Semin Perinatol* 1997;21(2):124–134.
2. Henshaw SK. Unintended pregnancy in the United States. *Fam Plann Perspect* 1998;30(1):24–29,46.

3. Broughton Pipkin F, Turner SR, Symonds EM. Possible risk with captopril in pregnancy: some animal data. *Lancet* 1980;1:1256.

4. Ferris TF, Weir EK. Effect of captopril on uterine blood flow and prostaglandin E synthesis in the pregnant rabbit. *J Clin Invest* 1983; 71:809–815.

5. Binder ND, Faber JJ. Effects of captopril on blood pressure, placental blood flow and uterine oxygen consumption in pregnant rabbits. *J Pharmacol Exp Ther* 1992;260:294–299.

6. De Moura R, Lopes MA. Effect of captopril on the human foetal placental circulation: an interaction with bradykinine and angiotensin I. *Br J Clin Pharmacol* 1995;39:497–501.

7. Woods LL. Role of angiotensin II and prostaglandins in the regulation of uteroplacental blood flow. *Am J Physiol* 1993;264(3 Pt 2):R584–590.

8. Centres for Disease Control and Prevention. Postmarketing surveillance for angiotensin-converting enzyme inhibitor use during the first trimester of pregnancy, United States, Canada and Israel, 1987–1995. *MMWR Morb Mortal Wkly Rep* 1997;46:240–242.

9. Piper JM, Ray WA, Rosa FW. Pregnancy outcome following exposure to angiotensin-converting enzyme inhibitors. *Obstet Gynecol* 1992;80(3 Pt 1): 429–432.

10. Kreft-Jais C, Plouin PF, Tchbroutsky C, et al. Angiotensin-converting enzyme inhibitors during pregnancy: a survey of 22 patients given captopril and nine given enalapril. *Br J Obstet Gynaecol* 1988;95:420–422.

11. Tabacova S, Little R, Tsong Y, et al. Adverse pregnancy outcomes associated with maternal enalapril antihypertensive treatment. *Pharmacoepidemiol Drug Saf* 2003;12(8):633–646.

12. Lip GY, Churchill D, Beevers M, et al. Angiotensin-converting-enzyme inhibitors in early pregnancy. *Lancet* 1997;350:1446–1447.

LOW-MOLECULAR-WEIGHT HEPARINS DURING PREGNANCY

Ariel Many, MD, MHA
Gideon Koren, MD, FRCPC

QUESTION

A few years ago I suffered from pulmonary emboli. My physician recommended I use dalteparin during this pregnancy although, during my previous pregnancy, I had received subcutaneous heparin injections three times daily. Is dalteparin the same as heparin?

Answer

Based on the best available evidence from mostly small prospective case series, retrospective reports, and placental perfusion studies, low-molecular-weight heparins (LMWHs), such as dalteparin, are a safe and convenient alternative to heparin during pregnancy for both mothers and fetuses.

Low-molecular-weight heparins have shorter polysaccharide chains and lower molecular weights than unfractionated heparin. Low-molecular-weight heparins are widely used, mainly for thromboprophylaxis. These agents are dalteparin (Fragmin), enoxaparin (Lovenox), certoparin, and a few other less popular preparations. The pharmacokinetic and pharmacodynamic characteristics of LMWHs are substantially different from those of unfractionated heparin.

In clinical practice, LMWHs are much easier and more convenient for patients and physicians to use compared with unfractionated heparin. This is due to their long half-life and few side effects. There is also no need for frequent monitoring of partial thromboplastin time.

INDICATIONS DURING PREGNANCY

There are several indications for anticoagulation treatment during pregnancy. Pregnancy and the postpartum period are especially thrombogenic. Whenever a condition requiring anticoagulation (e.g., a current or recent thromboembolic event) would be treated in non-pregnant patients, it should usually be treated in pregnant patients also. One exception is thromboprophylaxis for patients with heart-valve prostheses. Several reports, including one from the U.S. Food and Drug Administration,[1] recommend not using LMWH for these patients during pregnancy. Only heparin should be used (warfarin is teratogenic). Why LMWHs are less effective for patients with this condition is yet to be determined.

PREGNANCY-SPECIFIC INDICATIONS

Antiphospholipid syndrome (APS) is associated with adverse pregnancy outcomes. A few controlled trials suggest that a combination of heparin and acetylsalicylic acid (ASA) improves pregnancy outcomes in women with APS.[2,3]

In recent years, many reports have found an association between various thrombophilias and adverse pregnancy outcomes, such as preeclampsia, abruptio placentae, intrauterine growth restriction, recurrent abortions, and fetal death.[4-7] Only very limited hard data support use of LMWH for women with previous adverse pregnancy outcomes and thrombophilias. Nevertheless, offering these women anticoagulation therapy is relatively common. A recent article[8] has suggested that, for women with previous pregnancy loss and thrombophilia (namely factor V Leiden and prothrombin mutation), administration of LMWH rather than ASA improves pregnancy outcome. This new report might further increase use of LMWHs for women who have had previous adverse pregnancy outcomes.

DOSAGE AND MONITORING

In various reports, doses of dalteparin ranged from 2500 to 20,000 units in one or two subcutaneous (SC) injections daily. For enoxaparin, doses ranged from 20 to 120 mg/day divided into one or two SC injections daily.

There is no way of comparing dosage equivalences among the various LMWHs unit by unit, by pharmacokinetics, or by bioactivity. Testing anti-Xa levels will allow physicians to monitor LMWH levels 3 to 4 hours after administration. The importance and optimal frequency of monitoring anti-Xa levels during treatment with LMWH are still debatable.

SIDE EFFECTS

The most common side effects of heparin are bleeding, osteoporosis, and heparin-induced thrombocytopenia. The LMWHs have weaker interactions with platelets and inhibit bone formation less than unfractionated heparin. They also have higher bioavailability after SC administration, have a longer half-life, and are less bound to plasma proteins. All these factors make LMWHs less likely than heparin to cause side effects. Much less osteoporosis is seen with LMWH treatment. One recent study showed no difference in bone density until after pregnancy between women who had and had not been treated with LMWHs.[9,10] Heparin-induced thrombocytopenia is very rare with use of LMWH.

A common side effect reported is skin irritation at the injection site. This should not result in cessation of treatment.

TRANSFER TO FETUS AND MILK

An in vitro experimental study by Motherisk showed that LMWHs did not cross the placenta.[11] A clinical report, where LMWH was injected shortly before a late pregnancy termination, showed that anti-Xa was detected in the women but not in the fetuses, indicating no LMWH crossed the placenta.[12] In retrospective studies, no specific adverse fetal effects or teratogenicity were detected.[13] It should be noted that LMWHs are classified by the Food and Drug Administration as pregnancy category B (no evidence of adverse effects on humans). The concentration of LMWH in maternal milk was very low, more than 10 times lower than in maternal serum, and thus had no clinical significance.[12] Women treated with LMWHs can safely breastfeed.

REFERENCES

1. US Food and Drug Administration. FDA Med Watch. Rockville, Md: Food and Drug Administration; 2002. Available at: *http://www.fda.gov/medwat*. Accessed 2004 September 1.

2. Rai R, Cohen H, Dave M, et al. Controlled trial of aspirin and aspirin plus heparin in pregnant women with recurrent miscarriage associated with phospholipid antibodies (or antiphospholipid antibodies). *BMJ* 1997;314 (7076):253–257.

3. Duley L, Henderson-Smart D, Knight M, et al. Antiplatelet drugs for prevention of pre-eclampsia and its consequences: systematic review. *BMJ* 2001;322:329–333.

4. Dekker GA, de Vries JIP, Doelitzsch PM, et al. Underlying disorders associated with severe early-onset preeclampsia. *Am J Obstet Gynecol* 1995;173:1042–1048.

5. Kupferminc MJ, Eldor A, Steinman N, et al. Increased frequency of the genetic thrombophilia in women with complications of pregnancy. *N Engl J Med* 1999;340:9–13.

6. Martinelli I, Taioli E, Cetin I, et al. Mutations in coagulation factors in women with unexplained late fetal loss. *N Engl J Med* 2000;343: 1015–1018.

7. Many A, Elad R, Yaron Y, et al. Third-trimester unexplained intrauterine fetal death is associated with inherited thrombophilia. *Obstet Gynecol* 2002;99:684–687.

8. Gris JC, Mercier E, Quere I, et al. Low-molecular-weight heparin versus low-dose aspirin in women with one fetal loss and a constitutional thrombophilic disorder. *Blood* 2004;103:3695–3699.

9. Pettila V, Leinonen P, Markkola A, et al. Postpartum bone mineral density in women treated for thromboprophylaxis with unfractionated heparin or LMW heparin. *Thromb Haemost* 2002;87(2):182–186.

10. Carlin AJ, Farquharson RG, Quenby SM, et al. Prospective observational study of bone mineral density during pregnancy: low molecular weight heparin versus control. *Hum Reprod* 2004;19(5):1211–1214.

11. Boskovic B, Koren G. Placental transfer of drugs. In: Yaffe J, Aranda JU, eds. *Neonatal and Pediatric Pharmacology*. Philadelphia, Pa: Lippincot Williams and Wilkins; 2005. p. 136.

12. Dimitrakakis C, Papageorgiou P, Papageorgiou I, et al. Absence of transplacental passage of the low molecular weight heparin enoxaparin. *Haemostasis* 2000;30:243–248.

13. Richter C, Sitzmann J, Lang P, et al. Excretion of low molecular weight heparin in human milk. *Br J Clin Pharmacol* 2001;52(6):708–710.

CHAPTER 22

DRINKING ALCOHOL WHILE BREASTFEEDING: WILL IT HARM MY BABY?

Gideon Koren, MD, FRCPC
Myla Moretti, MSc

QUESTION

I recently delivered a healthy, full-term baby and am now breastfeeding exclusively. I abstained from drinking alcohol during my entire pregnancy and am wondering if drinking alcohol now would harm my nursing baby.

Answer

Nursing mothers who choose to drink alcohol during the postpartum period should carefully plan a breastfeeding schedule by storing milk before drinking and waiting for complete elimination of alcohol from their breast milk after drinking. Motherisk has created an algorithm to estimate how long it takes to eliminate alcohol from breast milk.

Ample evidence indicates that drinking alcohol during pregnancy poses a severe and avoidable risk to unborn babies. The risks of drinking alcohol while breastfeeding, however, are not well-defined. Currently, some mothers are still advised by physicians, nurses, lactation consultants, family members, and friends that it is all right to drink,[1] even though an acceptable level of alcohol in breast milk has never been established.

Alcohol consumed by a mother passes easily into her breast milk at concentrations similar to those found in her bloodstream. A nursing infant is actually exposed to only a fraction of the alcohol the mother ingests,[2] but infants detoxify alcohol in their first weeks of life at only half the rate of adults.[3]

Several proven or potential adverse effects of alcohol on suckling infants have been reported, even after exposure to only moderate levels: impaired motor development,[4] changes in sleep patterns,[5] decrease in milk intake,[6] and risk of hypoglycemia.[7] In addition, drinking large amounts of alcohol could affect lactating women's milk flow.[8,9]

Some report that beer aids milk production and that infants prefer alcohol-flavored breast milk. Even though beer increases maternal milk production and alcohol enhances its flavor, evidence indicates that the presence of alcohol in breast milk has an overall effect of decreasing infant consumption by 23%.[6] The underlying mechanism for this reduction is unknown.

At this time, there are no known benefits of exposing nursing infants to alcohol. Although occasional drinking while nursing has not been associated with overt harm to infants, the possibility of adverse effects has not been ruled out. Occasional drinking, however, does not warrant discontinuing breastfeeding, as the benefits of breastfeeding are extensive and well recognized.[10] Until a safe level of alcohol in breast milk is established, no alcohol in breast milk is safest for nursing babies. It is, therefore, prudent for mothers to delay breast-feeding their babies until alcohol is completely cleared from their breast milk.

Previous guidelines for determining the time needed to eliminate alcohol from breast milk were rough estimates based on number of drinks consumed. By also taking into account mother's weight, which affects milk-alcohol concentration, a more accurate estimate of how long a nursing mother should delay breastfeeding can be determined.

With pharmacokinetic modeling, the Motherisk team produced an algorithm to help breastfeeding mothers and their health care providers determine how long it takes to eliminate alcohol completely from breast milk (Table 22-1).[11] Time should be calculated from the beginning of drinking.

Because alcohol elimination follows zero-order kinetics, drinking water, resting, or "pumping and dumping" breast milk will not accelerate elimination.[12] Unlike urine, which stores substances in the bladder, alcohol is not trapped in breast milk, but is constantly removed as it diffuses back into the bloodstream.[2]

Mothers who choose to drink alcohol while breastfeeding should be aware of the documented effects on nursing infants. Carefully planning a breastfeeding schedule and waiting for complete alcohol clearance from breast milk can ensure that babies are not exposed to any alcohol.

TABLE 22-1
TIME FROM BEGINNING OF DRINKING UNTIL CLEARANCE OF ALCOHOL FROM BREAST MILK FOR WOMEN OF VARIOUS BODY WEIGHTS: ASSUMING ALCOHOL METABOLISM IS CONSTANT AT 15 MG/DL AND WOMAN IS OF AVERAGE HEIGHT (1.62 M [5'4"])

Mother's Weight kg (lb)	No. Of Drinks* (Hours : Minutes)											
	1	2	3	4	5	6	7	8	9	10	11	12
40.8 (90)	2:50	5:40	8:30	11:20	14:10	17:00	19:51	22:41				
43.1 (95)	2:46	5:32	8:19	11:05	13:52	16:38	19:25	22:11				
45.4 (100)	2:42	5:25	8:08	10:51	13:34	16:17	19:00	21:43				
47.6 (105)	2:39	5:19	7:58	10:38	13:18	15:57	18:37	21:16	23:56			
49.9 (110)	2:36	5:12	7:49	10:25	13:01	15:38	18:14	20:50	23:27			
52.2 (115)	2:33	5:06	7:39	10:12	12:46	15:19	17:52	20:25	22:59			
54.4 (120)	2:30	5:00	7:30	10:00	12:31	15:01	17:31	20:01	22:32			
56.7 (125)	2:27	4:54	7:22	9:49	12:16	14:44	17:11	19:38	22:06			
59.0 (130)	2:24	4:49	7:13	9:38	12:03	14:27	16:52	19:16	21:41			

kg (lb)											
61.2 (135)	2:21	4:43	7:05	9:27	11:49	14:11	16:33	18:55	21:17	23:39		
63.5 (140)	2:19	4:38	6:58	9:17	11:37	13:56	16:15	18:35	20:54	23:14		
65.8 (145)	2:16	4:33	6:50	9:07	11:24	13:41	15:58	18:15	20:32	22:49		
68.0 (150)	2:14	4:29	6:43	8:58	11:12	13:27	15:41	17:56	20:10	22:25		
70.3 (155)	2:12	4:24	6:36	8:48	11:01	13:13	15:25	17:37	19:49	22:02		
72.6 (160)	2:10	4:20	6:30	8:40	10:50	13:00	15:10	17:20	19:30	21:40	23:50	
74.8 (165)	2:07	4:15	6:23	8:31	10:39	12:47	14:54	17:02	19:10	21:18	23:50	
77.1 (170)	2:05	4:11	6:17	8:23	10:28	12:34	14:40	16:46	18:51	20:57	23:03	
79.3 (175)	2:03	4:07	6:11	8:14	10:18	12:22	14:26	16:29	18:33	20:37	22:40	
81.6 (180)	2:01	4:03	6:05	8:07	10:08	12:10	14:12	16:14	18:15	20:17	22:19	
83.9 (185)	1:59	3:59	5:59	7:59	9:59	11:59	13:59	15:59	17:58	19:58	21:58	23:58
86.2 (190)	1:58	3:56	5:54	7:52	9:50	11:48	13:46	15:44	17:42	19:40	21:38	23:36
88.5 (195)	1:56	3:52	5:48	7:44	9:41	11:37	13:33	15:29	17:26	19:22	21:18	23:14

(Continued)

TABLE 22-1
TIME FROM BEGINNING OF DRINKING UNTIL CLEARANCE OF ALCOHOL FROM BREAST MILK FOR WOMEN OF VARIOUS BODY WEIGHTS: ASSUMING ALCOHOL METABOLISM IS CONSTANT AT 15 MG/DL AND WOMAN IS OF AVERAGE HEIGHT (1.62 M [5'4"]) (*Continued*)

Mother's Weight kg (lb)	No. Of Drinks* (Hours : Minutes)											
	1	2	3	4	5	6	7	8	9	10	11	12
90.7 (200)	1:54	3:49	5:43	7:38	9:32	11:27	13:21	15:16	17:10	19:05	20:59	22:54
93.0 (205)	1:52	3:45	5:38	7:31	9:24	11:17	13:09	15:02	16:55	18:48	20:41	22:34
95.3 (210)	1:51	3:42	5:33	7:24	9:16	11:07	12:58	14:49	16:41	18:32	20:23	22:14

* **1 drink** = 340 g (12 oz) of 5% beer, or 141.75 g (5 oz) of 11% wine, or 42.53 g (1.5 oz) of 40% liquor.

Example no. 1: For a 40.8 kg (90 lb) woman who consumed three drinks in 1 hour, it would take 8 hours, 30 minutes for there to be no alcohol in her breast milk, but for a 95.3 kg (210 lb) woman drinking the same amount, it would take 5 hours, 33 minutes.

Example no. 2: For a 63.5 kg (140 lb) woman drinking four beers starting at 8:00 PM, it would take 9 hours, 17 minutes for there to be no alcohol in her breast milk (i.e., until 5:17 AM).

REFERENCES

1. Menella JA. Infant's suckling response to the flavor of alcohol in mother's milk. *Alcohol Clin Exp Res* 1997;21:581–585.
2. Lawton ME. Alcohol in breast milk. *Aust N Z J Obstet Gynaecol* 1985; 25:71–73.
3. Abel EL. Pharmacology of alcohol relating to pregnancy and lactation. Buffalo, NY: Plenum Press; 1984:29–45.
4. Little RE, Anderson KW, Ervin CH, Worthington-Roberts B, Clarren SK. Maternal alcohol use during breastfeeding and infant mental and motor development at one year. *N Engl J Med* 1989;321:425–430.
5. Mennella JA, Gerrish CJ. Effects of exposure to alcohol in mother's milk on infant sleep. *Pediatrics* 1998;101:E2.
6. Mennella JA, Beauchamp GK. The transfer of alcohol to human milk. Effects on flavor and the infant's behavior. *N Engl J Med* 1991;325: 981–985.
7. Lamminpaa A. Alcohol intoxication in childhood and adolescence. *Alcohol Alcohol* 1995;30:5–12.
8. Cobo E. Effect of different doses of ethanol on the milk-ejection reflex in lactating women. *Am J Obstet Gynecol* 1973;115:817–821.
9. Coiro V, Alboni A, Gramellini D, et al. Inhibition by ethanol of the oxytocin response to breast stimulation in normal women and the role of endogenous opioids. *Acta Endocrinol* 1992;126:213–216.
10. American Academy of Pediatrics. Work Group on Breastfeeding. Breastfeeding and the use of human milk. Work Group on Breastfeeding. American Academy of Pediatrics. *Pediatrics* 1997;100:1035–1039.
11. Ho E, Collantes A, Kapur BM, et al. Alcohol and breastfeeding: calculation of time to zero level in milk. *Biol Neonate* 2001;80:219–222.
12. Anderson PO. The galactopharmacopedia, alcohol and breastfeeding. *J Hum Lact* 1995;11:321–323.

MULTIVITAMIN SUPPLEMENTS FOR PREGNANT WOMEN: NEW INSIGHTS

Alejandro A. Nava-Ocampo, MD
Gideon Koren, MD, FRCPC

QUESTION

One of my patients is planning pregnancy and has started taking multivitamin supplements. She is experiencing gastric discomfort. What are the alternatives?

Answer

Gastric discomfort is usually related to iron intake; pregnant women could use supplements with less iron. Pregnant women need 0.4 to 1.0 mg of folic acid daily. If they have a family history of neural tube defects (NTDs), insulin-dependent diabetes mellitus, or epilepsy, or are currently taking valproic acid, carbamazepine, or antifolates (e.g., sulfonamides), they are at intermediate-to-high risk of having babies with NTDs and need 4.0 to 5.0 mg of folic acid daily.

Prenatal multivitamins are recommended before and during pregnancy to prevent iron-deficiency anemia and NTDs.[1-3] A range of prenatal supplements are available; most meet the required dietary allowance for pregnant women.

Some patients have very low tolerance of iron because they have morning sickness, which is experienced by 50% to 80% of pregnant women.[4] A new twice-a-day prenatal multivitamin supplement (PregVit) might be an appropriate alternative for women unable to tolerate the side effects of ingesting iron at high doses. The morning tablet contains 35 mg of iron, almost 50% less than is in most prenatal multivitamins. Calcium is provided in the night tablet so that it does not interfere with the absorption of iron, which is why the lower dose of iron is adequate.[5,6] A recent study at the Motherisk program showed that patients absorbed similar amounts of iron from PregVit and another widely used prenatal supplement.

Even today, following folate fortification of flour, about half of Canadian women have folate levels below the protective 900 nM and thus are at increased risk of having babies with NTDs.[7] Folic acid supplementation is especially important before closure of the neural tube at approximately 28 days' gestation (iron becomes more important during the second and third trimesters). Folic acid might be beneficial throughout the first trimester in preventing other malformations also.[8]

Women who have a family history of NTDs, insulin-dependent diabetes mellitus, or epilepsy, or are currently taking valproic acid, carbamazepine, or antifolates (e.g., sulfonamides) are at intermediate-to-high risk of having babies with NTDs. These women need 4 to 5 mg of folic acid daily starting before they become pregnant.

New and potentially important findings were recently reported in an analysis of all published folic acid dose-level studies. Results demonstrated that to achieve the needed serum concentration of 900 nM, 5 mg of folic acid is required daily. This dose, rather than the previously recommended 0.4 to 1.0 mg dose, could prevent 85% of folate-dependent NTDs.[9] The main concern with this high dose of folic acid is that it could mask vitamin B_{12}' deficiency pernicious anemia. Making a general recommendation for higher folate supplementation must await in-depth analysis of the effects of the low folate fortification instituted in the United States and Canada in 1997 to 1998.

Prenatal multivitamins contain iron and calcium, both of which are potent inhibitors of absorption of levothyroxine.[10,11] A recent study found that doses of levothyroxine do not need to be modified if prenatal multivitamins are taken 4 hours after ingestion of levothyroxine.[12] Concomitant ingestion of iron causes marked decreases in the bioavailability of a variety of drugs.[13] The major mechanism of these drug interactions is the formation of iron-drug complexes.

Finally, recent studies suggest that supplementation of prenatal vitamins may prevent other malformations, including cardiac, limb, and central nervous system (CNS).[14]

REFERENCES

1. Beaton GH. Iron needs during pregnancy: do we need to rethink our targets Am J Clin Nutr 2000;72(Suppl 1):265–271S.
2. MRC Vitamin Study Research Group. Prevention of neural tube defects: results of the Medical Research Council Vitamin Study. Lancet 1991;338: 131–137.
3. Czeizel AE, Dudas I. Prevention of the first occurrence of neural-tube defects by periconceptional vitamin supplementation. N Engl J Med 1992;327:1832–1835.
4. Koren G, Boskovic R, Hard M, et al. Motherisk-PUQE (pregnancy-unique quantification of emesis and nausea) scoring system for nausea and vomiting of pregnancy. Am J Obstet Gynecol 2002;186(Suppl 5): S228–S231.
5. Bendich A. Calcium supplementation and iron status of females. Nutrition 2001;17:46–51.
6. Zijp IM, Korver O, Tijburg LB. Effect of tea and other dietary factors on iron absorption. Crit Rev Food Sci Nutr 2000;40:371–398.
7. Kapur B, Soldin OP, Koren G. Potential prevention of neural tube defects by assessment of women of childbearing age through monitoring of folate. Ther Drug Monit 2002;24:628–630.
8. French AE, Grant R, Weitzman S, et al. Folic acid food fortification is associated with a decline in neuroblastoma. Clin Pharmacol Ther 2003; 74:288–294.
9. Wald NJ, Law MR, Morris JK, et al. Quantifying the effect of folic acid. Lancet 2001;358:2069–2073.
10. Campbell NR, Hasinoff BB, Stalts H, et al. Ferrous sulfate reduces thyroxine efficacy in patients with hypothyroidism. Ann Intern Med 1992; 117:1010–1013.
11. Singh N, Singh PN, Hershman JM. Effect of calcium carbonate on the absorption of levothyroxine. JAMA 2000;283:2822–2825.
12. Chopra IJ, Baber K. Treatment of primary hypothyroidism during pregnancy: is there an increase in thyroxine dose requirement in pregnancy? Metabolism 2003;52:122–128.
13. Campbell NR, Hasinoff BB. Iron supplements: a common cause of drug interactions. Br J Clin Pharmacol 1991;31:251–255.
14. Goh I, Bollano E, Einarson TR, Koren G. Prenatal multivitamin supplementation and rates of congenital malformation: A meta-analysis. J Obstet Gynaecol Can 2006;28:680–689.

FOLIC ACID AND NEURAL TUBE DEFECTS: GOOD NEWS AT LAST!

Gideon Koren, MD, FRCPC

QUESTION

I read last year that Canada has followed the United States in fortifying flour with folic acid to prevent neural tube defects (NTDs). Do we know yet whether this strategy is working?

Answer

In Canada, flour is fortified with folic acid to a level of 0.15 mg/100 g. Although a mandatory date was set for November 1, 1998, most if not all companies implemented the change on or before January 1, 1998. Recent figures from the United States, where the deadline for fortification was January 1998, show that by March 1999, mean folate levels in flour doubled, substantially decreasing the risk for NTDs.

Two large randomized, blinded controlled studies have documented the effect of folic acid supplementation before pregnancy on prevention of NTDs.[1,2] On average, Canadian women consume 200 mg/day of folic acid; 400 mg/day are needed to prevent a first NTD.[3] Because the neural tube is fused within the first month of pregnancy, folic acid supplementation later than that (e.g., at 2 or 3 months' gestation) does not prevent NTDs. Because at least half of all pregnancies are unplanned, many women are likely to find out they have conceived too late for an intervention with folic acid to have a therapeutic effect. Because of this, the only effective solution to preventing folic-acid preventable NTDs is to fortify a commonly used food staple.

In January 1998, the U.S. Food and Drug Administration put into effect a new regulation that enforced adding 140 mg of folic acid per 100g of flour (in addition to other vitamins already added). This level of fortification would, it was believed, increase "average" women's folic acid intake by 80 to 100 mg/day. Researchers acknowledged that this level might not be high enough to prevent all preventable cases of NTDs.[4] In May 1999, Jacques and colleagues[5] reported the effect of this fortification, as measured in March 1999, using patients followed in the Framingham Heart Study.

Among subjects not using vitamin supplements, serum concentrations of folic acid increased from 4.6 to 10.0 ng/mL (11 to 23 nmol/L) (P <.001) between prefortification and postfortification visits. The prevalence of low folate concentrations (< 3 ng/mL) decreased from 22% to 1.7% (P <.001).

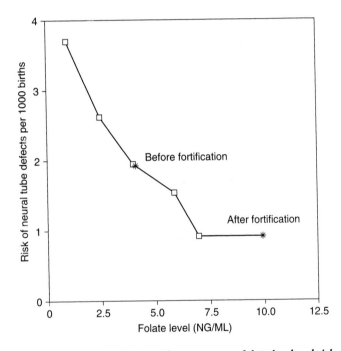

FIGURE 24-1 *Relationship between serum folate level and risk of neural tube defects (NTDs):* The increase in folate levels in the United States decreased the risk of NTDs by more than half. *(Adapted from Daly LE, Kirke PM, Molloy A, et al. Folate levels and neural tube defects: implications for prevention. JAMA 1995;274: 1698–1702. With additional data from Jacques PF, Selhub J, Bostom AG, et al. The effect of folic acid fortification on plasma folate and total homocysteine concentrations. N Engl J Med 1999;340:1449–1454)*

To put this important result in the context of risk for NTDs, we reviewed the concentration-response curve of serum folate with NTD risk per 1000 births established by Daly et al..[6] Based on this curve, the risk of NTDs would have decreased from 2 to 0.9 cases per 1000 births (Fig. 24-1[5,6]). In Canada, this would mean a reduction from 800 cases to 360 cases a year, although we should be cautious in extrapolating Irish figures to those in North America because North America's population is more heterogenous in terms of racial origins.

We must await new statistics on changes in serum folate concentrations in Canada after fortification. It is conceivable that a 30% to 40% decrease in NTDs could be expected even with the relatively low level of fortification.

REFERENCES

1. Wald N, Sneddon J, Densem J, et al. MRC vitamin Study Research Group. Prevention of neural tube defects: results of the MRC Vitamin Study. *Lancet* 1991;338:131–137.
2. Czeizel AE, Dudas I. Prevention of the first occurrence of neural tube defects by periconceptional vitamin supplementation. *N Engl J Med* 1992; 327:1832–1835.
3. O'Connor DL. The folate status of Canadian women. In: Koren G, ed.. *Folic acid for the prevention of neural tube defects*. Toronto, Ont: The Motherisk Program; 1995. p. 73–87.
4. Oakley GP Jr. Eat right and take a multivitamin. *N Engl J Med* 1998;338: 1060–1061.
5. Jacques PF, Selhub J, Bostom AG, et al. The effect of folic acid fortification on plasma folate and total homocysteine concentrations. *N Engl J Med* 1999;340:1449–1454.
6. Daly LE, Kirke PN, Molloy A, et al. Folate levels and neural tube defects: implications for prevention. *JAMA* 1995;274:1698–1702.

CHAPTER 25

SAFETY OF GADOLINIUM DURING PREGNANCY

Facundo Garcia-Bournissen, MD
Alon Shrim, MD
Gideon Koren, MD, FRCPC

QUESTION

A pregnant patient who underwent magnetic resonance imaging (MRI) because of an acute abdomen, was told that MRI contrast agents (i.e., gadolinium-based contrast agents) are contraindicated during pregnancy. What is the risk to her baby?

Answer

Current radiology practices and recommendations discourage the use of gadolinium-based contrast agents during pregnancy because their safety for the fetus has not yet been proven. In line, however, with the European Society of Radiology guidelines and based on the available evidence, gadolinium-based contrast agents appear to be safe in pregnancy. Gadolinium use should be considered when the diagnostic study is important for the health of the mother.

MRI is considered safe during pregnancy, as magnetic energy has been shown not to be harmful for the developing fetus.[1,2]

On the other hand, most radiology service providers consider gadolinium-based contrast agents for MRI (e.g., gadopentetate, gadodiamide, gadolinium DPTA, gadoterate meglumine) to be relatively or absolutely contraindicated during pregnancy; these paramagnetic agents are not recommended by the Food and Drug Administration because they cross the placenta and their long-term effects are unknown. All pregnant patients are expected to consult their obstetricians before undergoing MRI examination.

Gadolinium-based contrast agents are excreted almost exclusively by the kidneys through glomerular filtration. Their volume of distribution is equal to the volume of extracellular water, and binding to plasma proteins is negligible. These agents possess a very high safety index in human beings.[3]

Although there have not been any long-term animal studies to evaluate the carcinogenic potential of gadolinium-based contrast agents, no carcinogenic or mutagenic effects have been observed and no teratogenic or other long-term effects occurred in mice exposed in utero to gadolinium-based contrast agents.[4–7] Pregnant mice exposed to MRI with and without gadolinium had no differences in litter size, number of live offspring, fetal weight, morphology, or development, compared with unexposed controls.[4]

Gadolinium-based contrast agents have been detected in the placenta in animals and human beings.[8–10] In women during the second and third trimesters of pregnancy, uptake of gadolinium-based contrast agents by the placenta was sufficient for MRI imaging.[11,12] These agents have also been observed in animals, and occasionally in human beings, to cross the placenta into the fetal circulation and to be excreted by the fetal kidneys, appearing in the fetal bladder only minutes after administration to the mother.[3,13,14] Gadolinium-based contrast agents are believed to diffuse from the fetus back to the mother, given the high clearance rate observed in fetal rats.[15]

INADVERTENT EXPOSURE

Inadvertent human exposure during the first trimester of pregnancy has not been associated with adverse effects in the fetus.[16,17] Reports on use of gadolinium-based contrast agents during the second or third trimester are not rare,[10–13,18] underscoring the usefulness of these agents in diagnosing various conditions. No harm to the fetus has been documented in these circumstances.

GUIDELINES

The European Society of Radiology has issued a guideline[19] discussing gadolinium use during pregnancy. Their conclusion is that gadolinium is probably safe during pregnancy, as excessive quantities are not expected to cross the placenta or to be toxic to the fetus if they do.[19]

These guidelines also state that, given that gadolinium is mainly distributed in extracellular water and rapidly eliminated by the kidney, in the unlikely event that some gadolinium reached the baby, it would be rapidly eliminated into urine.[19]

CONCLUSION

Current radiology practices and recommendations discourage the use of gadolinium-based contrast agents during pregnancy because their safety for the fetus has not been proven. Yet available evidence suggests it is unlikely that these compounds have an adverse effect on the developing fetus; therefore, their use should not be limited, particularly given the important clinical reasons for MRI examinations during pregnancy (e.g., to rule out serious abdominal diseases).

REFERENCES

1. De Wilde JP, Rivers AW, Price DL. A review of the current use of magnetic resonance imaging in pregnancy and safety implications for the fetus. Prog Biophys Mol Biol 2005;87:335–353.
2. Nagayama M, Watanabe Y, Okumura A, et al. Fast MR imaging in obstetrics. Radiographics 2002;22:563–582.
3. Shellock FG, Kanal E. Safety of magnetic resonance imaging contrast agents. J Magn Reson Imaging 1999;10:477–484.
4. Rofsky NM, Pizzarello DJ, Weinreb JC, et al. Effect on fetal mouse development of exposure to MR imaging and gadopentetate dimeglumine. J Magn Reson Imaging 1994;4:805–807.
5. Soltys RA. Summary of preclinical safety evaluation of gadoteridol injection. Invest Radiol 1992;27(Suppl 1):S7–S11.
6. Morisetti A, Bussi S, Tirone P, et al. Toxicological safety evaluation of gadobenate dimeglumine 0.5 M solution for injection (MultiHance), a new magnetic resonance imaging contrast medium. J Comput Assist Tomogr 1999;23(Suppl 1):S207–S217.
7. Wible JH Jr, Galen KP, Wojdyla JK. Cardiovascular effects caused by rapid administration of gadoversetamide injection in anesthetized dogs. Invest Radiol 2001;36:292–298.
8. Salomon LJ, Siauve N, Balvay D, et al. Placental perfusion MR imaging with contrast agents in a mouse model. Radiology 2005;235:73–80.
9. Lam G, Kuller J, McMahon M. Use of magnetic resonance imaging and ultrasound in the antenatal diagnosis of placenta accreta. J Soc Gynecol Investig 2002;9:37–40.
10. Palacios Jaraquemada JM, Bruno C. Gadolinium-enhanced MR imaging in the differential diagnosis of placenta accreta and placenta percreta. Radiology 2000;216:610–611.

11. Marcos HB, Semelka RC, Worawattanakul S. Normal placenta: gadolinium-enhanced dynamic MR imaging. *Radiology* 1997;205:493–496.

12. Spencer JA, Tomlinson AJ, Weston MJ, et al. Early report: comparison of breath-hold MR excretory urography, Doppler ultrasound and isotope renography in evaluation of symptomatic hydronephrosis in pregnancy. *Clin Radiol* 2000;55:446–453.

13. Novak Z, Thurmond AS, Ross PL, et al. Gadolinium-DTPA transplacental transfer and distribution in fetal tissue in rabbits. *Invest Radiol* 1993;28: 828–830.

14. Chapon C, Franconi F, Roux J, et al. Prenatal evaluation of kidney function in mice using dynamic contrast-enhanced magnetic resonance imaging. *Anat Embryol* (Berl) 2005;209:263–267.

15. Okazaki O, Murayama N, Masubuchi N, et al. Placental transfer and milk secretion of gadodiamide injection in rats. *Arzneimittelforschung* 1996;46: 83–86.

16. Barkhof F, Heijboer RJ, Algra PR. Inadvertent i.v. administration of gadopentetate dimeglumine during early pregnancy. *AJR Am J Roentgenol* 1992;158:1171.

17. Shoenut JP, Semelka RC, Silverman R, et al. MRI in the diagnosis of Crohn's disease in two pregnant women. *J Clin Gastroenterol* 1993;17:244–247.

18. Leyendecker JR, Gorengaut V, Brown JJ. MR imaging of maternal diseases of the abdomen and pelvis during pregnancy and the immediate postpartum period. *Radiographics* 2004;24:1301–1316.

19. Webb JA, Thomsen HS, Morcos SK. The use of iodinated and gadolinium contrast media during pregnancy and lactation. *Eur Radiol* 2005;15: 1234–1240.

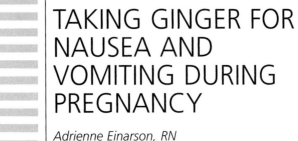

CHAPTER 26

TAKING GINGER FOR NAUSEA AND VOMITING DURING PREGNANCY

Adrienne Einarson, RN
Gideon Koren MD, FRCPC

QUESTION

Many of my patients prefer to use natural or herbal medicines, such as ginger, before taking drugs to treat nausea and vomiting of pregnancy. Is there evidence that ginger is safe to use during pregnancy? Is it effective?

Answer

Although ginger is used in many cultures to treat the symptoms of nausea and vomiting, no trials have established its safety for use during pregnancy. On the other hand, its efficacy has been documented in two randomized, blinded controlled trials.

Although nausea and vomiting of pregnancy (NVP) can affect up to 80% of all pregnant women,[1] it is largely ignored in medical research and in development of new treatments. Even when the condition is mild, symptoms can cause considerable distress and temporary disability.[2] Our research team at the Motherisk Program is one of very few groups to focus on treatment of NVP. In an attempt to improve the lives of women with NVP, we try to investigate the optimal treatment modalities.

Despite the fact that there is safe and effective pharmacologic treatment for NVP, many women and their physicians are still cautious and often fearful of taking drugs during pregnancy. Occasionally, lack of treatment leads to severe hyperemesis and results in hospitalization and rehydration with intravenous fluids. This has great emotional and financial costs.

Many women try alternative therapies for NVP that range from herbal products to homeopathic drugs to acupressure or acupuncture. These therapies seem attractive due to their natural status. Nonpharmacologic interventions, such as advice on diet and lifestyle changes, are often recommended before physicians discuss use of medication. The drug of choice in Canada for treating NVP is vitamin B_6 and doxylamine succinate (Diclectin). Other treatments, such as phenothiazines,[3] antihistamines,[3,4] and metoclopramide,[3,5] are also used.

Ginger has been one of the most widely used treatments for NVP, despite the fact that there are few data on either its safety or efficacy. A survey on management of NVP sent out to obstetricians and gynecologists in the United States found that 51.8% of respondents recommended ginger for treatment of moderate nausea.[6] We surveyed 500 women suffering from severe NVP and found that 17% of them preferred nondrug treatments, such as ginger, to treat their symptoms.[2]

The efficacy of ginger is thought to be due to its aromatic, carminative, and absorbent properties.[7] Two randomized controlled trials in the literature report on the efficacy of ginger for NVP.[8,9] The first was a small crossover trial with 27 women admitted to hospital for treatment of hyperemesis gravidarum. They were given 250-mg ginger capsules four times daily for 4 days. This was followed by a 2-day washout period and a second 4-day period during which they were given 250-mg placebo capsules. The severity and relief of symptoms before and after each period were evaluated. A significant reduction in the symptoms of hyperemesis, measured as degree of nausea and number of vomiting attacks ($P = .035$), was observed with the ginger treatment.

A recent parallel control trial of 70 women randomized 35 of them to treatment with 250-mg ginger capsules and 35 to 250-mg placebo capsules four times daily for 4 days. Subjects graded the severity of nausea using visual analog scales and recorded the number of vomiting episodes. A five-item Likert scale was used to assess the severity of their NVP symptoms. Both symptoms of nausea ($P = .014$) and number of vomiting episodes ($P < .001$) decreased significantly with ginger. Likert scale scores showed that 28 of 35 in the ginger group experienced improvement in nausea symptoms compared with only 10 of 35 in the placebo group ($P < .001$).

Until recently, research has not adequately addressed whether ginger is safe for developing fetuses. Animal studies have shown ginger to be a potent thromboxane synthetase inhibitor; it could affect testosterone receptor binding and sex steroid differentiation in the fetal brain.[10] In a recent prospective controlled study by Motherisk, use of ginger was not associated with increased teratogenic risk.

Nausea and vomiting of pregnancy is a serious condition that should be treated appropriately. Ginger is an effective remedy that is used in many traditional cultures and frequently mentioned in the literature as a treatment for nausea and vomiting with no evidence to suggest it is teratogenic.

REFERENCES

1. Gadsby R, Barnie-Ashead AM, Jagger C. A prospective study of nausea and vomiting during pregnancy. *Br J Gen Pract* 1993;43:245–248.
2. Chandra K. *Development of a Health-Related Quality of Life Instrument for Nausea and Vomiting of Pregnancy.* Toronto, Ont: Department of Pharmacology, University of Toronto; 2000. Unpublished.
3. Mazzotta P, Magee L. A risk-benefit assessment of pharmacological and nonpharmacological treatments for nausea and vomiting of pregnancy. *Drugs* 2000;59:781–800.
4. Seto A, Einarson T, Koren G. Pregnancy outcome following first trimester exposure to antihistamines: meta-analysis. *Am J Perinatol* 1997;14: 119–124.
5. Einarson A, Koren G, Bergman U. Nausea and vomiting in pregnancy: a comparative study. *Eur J Obstet Gynecol Reprod Biol* 1998;76:1–3.
6. Power ML, Holzman GB, Schulkin J. A survey on the management of nausea and vomiting in pregnancy by obstetricians/gynecologists. *Prim Care Update Ob Gyns* 2001;8:69–72.
7. Murphy PA. Alternative therapies for NVP. *Obstet Gynecol* 1998;91: 149–155.
8. Fischer-Rasmussen WF, Kajaer S, Dahl C, et al. Ginger treatment of hyperemesis gravidarum. *Eur J Obstet Gynecol Reprod Biol* 1990;38: 19–24.
9. Vutyavanich T, Kraisarin T, Ruangsri R. Ginger for nausea and vomiting in pregnancy: randomized, double-masked, placebo-controlled trial. *Obstet Gynecol* 2001;97:577–582.
10. Backon J. Ginger, inhibition of thromboxane synthetase and stimulation of prostacyclin: relevance for medicine and psychiatry. *Med Hypoth* 1986; 20:271–278.
11. Portnoi G, Chng LA, Karimi-Tabesh L, Koren G, Tan MP, Einarson A: Prospective comparative study of the safety and effectiveness of ginger for the treatment of nausea and vomiting in pregnancy. *Am J Obstet Gynecol* 2003;189:1374–7.

CHAPTER 27

OCCUPATIONAL EXPOSURE TO INHALED ANESTHETIC: IS IT A CONCERN FOR PREGNANT WOMEN?

Samar R. Shuhaiber, MSc
Gideon Koren, MD, FRCPC

QUESTION

Two of my pregnant patients are exposed to inhaled anesthetic on the job. One is an anesthetist, and the other is a veterinarian. They have both expressed concern about this exposure. How should I advise them?

Answer

Occupational exposure to waste anesthetic gas is not associated with increased risk of major malformations. Risk of spontaneous abortion might be slightly increased, however. This risk can be reduced, if not eliminated, by good gas scavenging systems.

Currently, 854 anesthetists practise in Ontario; 25% of them are women, and 46% of those are of childbearing age, according to the Ontario Physician Human Resources Data Centre at McMaster University in Hamilton, Ont. The College of Veterinarians of Ontario indicates there are 2745 practising veterinarians in the province; approximately 45% of them are women.[1] Although there are numerous studies in the medical literature on the effects of occupational exposure to waste anesthetic gas (WAG) on the reproductive system, to date there have been no prospective controlled studies.

There are more data on the effects of exposure to WAG on pregnant women working in operating rooms than on those working in the veterinary field. Most existing evidence does not associate occupational exposure to WAG with increased risk of congenital malformations.[2-11]

ASSOCIATION WITH SPONTANEOUS ABORTION

A recent meta-analysis showed, however, that occupational exposure to WAG is associated with increased risk of spontaneous abortion (relative risk 1.48, 95% confidence interval[CI] 1.4 to 1.58).[12] This meta-analysis included 19 studies of various designs with anesthetists, operating-room physicians and nurses, dental assistants, operating-room workers, hospital workers, health workers, and veterinarians and veterinary assistants as subjects. Most of the studies included in the meta-analysis were conducted before WAG scavenging had become a legal requirement, and none of the studies attempted to establish a relationship between amount of exposure and magnitude of risk of spontaneous abortion. The most important limitation is that all the studies were retrospective.

VETERINARY WORK

In the veterinary field, Johnson et al.[13] have shown that even though the odds ratio (OR) for spontaneous abortion after exposure to WAG among female veterinarians and female veterinary assistants was greater than 1.0 when adjusted for use of diagnostic x-ray machines, it did not reach statistical significance. Schenker et al.[14] demonstrated that rates of spontaneous abortion and low birth weight infants were statistically similar among female veterinarians and lawyers.

It is a misconception that concentrations of WAG are much greater in veterinary facilities than in human operating rooms. Ward and Byland[15] measured WAG levels of 2 parts per million (ppm) in veterinary facilities and 10 ppm in human hospitals. Even though average room size in veterinary practice is smaller, operating times are short, and doors of veterinary surgery rooms are normally left open to allow technicians to work concurrently in other rooms.[15] In addition, veterinary staff spend only a small portion of their working time performing surgeries.[15] Despite all these factors, the level of WAG in veterinary facilities depends primarily on the presence of gas scavenging systems, good anesthetic practices, and periodic examination and maintenance of anesthetic machines.

NITROUS OXIDE

Most of the studies did not differentiate between the various inhaled anesthetics because subjects were anesthetists, operating room staff, or hospital staff who were exposed to mixtures of gases. A few studies examined the association between occupational exposure to nitrous oxide and spontaneous abortion among dental assistants and midwives.

Studies on dental staff's exposure to WAG had conflicting results. Cohen et al.[16] showed an increased risk of spontaneous abortion among dental assistants exposed to nitrous oxide (P value not reported). Heidam,[17] on the other hand, showed no increased risk for dental assistants either practicing in private clinics or working in dental school services (OR 0.4). Last, Rowland et al.[18] demonstrated increased risk of spontaneous abortion among dental assistants exposed to nitrous oxide for 3 or more hours weekly in places without scavenging systems.

A study of Swedish midwives exposed to nitrous oxide in more than 50% of deliveries showed no increased risk of spontaneous abortion (OR 0.95). The effect of WAG scavenging was excluded because many midwives were unsure about whether such equipment had been present in the delivery rooms.[19]

These findings clearly indicate that the question of whether occupational exposure to nitrous oxide increases risk of spontaneous abortion is complicated. The answer depends on the field in which nitrous oxide is being used because this dictates duration of exposure and anesthetic techniques used.

CONCLUSION

Pregnant patients should aim to minimize their exposure to WAG by always using scavenging systems, by periodically testing anesthetic machines for gas leaks, and by not emptying or filling vaporizers. We also recommend good anesthetic techniques including use of cuffed endotracheal tubes whenever feasible, avoiding use of anesthetic chambers or masks (veterinary staff), and maintaining connections between animals and anesthetic machines such that animals breathe pure oxygen for a few minutes once vaporizers are switched off (veterinary staff). Monitoring WAG is possible through air sampling, dosimeter badges, and portable infrared analyzers, but monitoring is costly and, therefore, not routinely practiced.

REFERENCES

1. Osborne D. Changing gender demographics. *J Ont Vet Med Assoc* 1999;18(5):15.
2. Lauwerys R, Siddons M, Misson CB, et al. Anaesthetic health hazards among Belgian nurses and physicians. *Int Arch Occup Environ Health* 1981;48(2):195–203.
3. Rosenberg PH, Vanttinen H. Occupational hazards to reproduction and health in anaesthetists and paediatricians. *Acta Anaesthesiol Scand* 1978;22:202–207.
4. Ad Hoc Committee on the effect of trace anesthetics on health of operating room personnel, American Society of Anesthesiologists. Occupational disease among operating room personnel: national study. *Anesthesiology* 1974;41(4):321–340.
5. Tomlin PJ. Health problems of anaesthetists and their families in the West Midlands. *BMJ* 1979;1:779–784.
6. Spence AA, Cohen EN, Brown BW Jr, et al. Occupational hazards for operating room' based physicians. Analysis of data from the United States and the United Kingdom. *JAMA* 1977;238:955–959.
7. Hemminki K, Kyyrönen P, Lindbohm ML. Spontaneous abortions and malformations in the offspring of nurses exposed to anaesthetic gases, cytostatic drugs, and other potential hazards in hospitals, based on registered information of outcome. *J Epidemiol Community Health* 1985; 39(2):141–147.
8. Sass-Kortsak AM, Purdham JT, Bozek PR, et al. Exposure of hospital operating room personnel to potentially harmful environmental agents. *Am Ind Hyg Assoc J* 1992;53(3):203–209.
9. Axelsson G, Rylander R. Exposure to anaesthetic gases and spontaneous abortion: response bias in a postal questionnaire study. *Int J Epidemiol* 1982;11:250–256.
10. Rosenberg P, Kirves A. Miscarriages among operating theatre staff. *Acta Anaesthesiol Scand Suppl* 1973;53:37–42.
11. Cohen EN, Bellville JW, Brown BW Jr. Anesthesia, pregnancy, and miscarriage: a study of operating room nurses and anesthetists. *Anesthesiology* 1971;35(4):343–347.
12. Boivin J. Risk of spontaneous abortion in women occupationally exposed to anaesthetic gases: a meta-analysis. *Occup Environ Med* 1997;54:541–548.
13. Johnson JA, Buchan RM, Reif JS. Effect of waste gas and vapor exposure on reproductive outcome in veterinary personnel. *Am Ind Hyg Assoc J* 1987;48(1):62–66.
14. Schenker MB, Samuels SJ, Green RS, et al. Adverse reproductive outcomes among female veterinarians. *Am J Epidemiol* 1990;132:96–106.
15. Ward GS, Byland RR. Concentration of halothane in veterinary operating and treatment rooms. *J Am Vet Med Assoc* 1982;180:174–177.
16. Cohen EN, Gift HC, Brown BW, et al. Occupational disease in dentistry and chronic exposure to trace anesthetic gases. *J Am Dent Assoc* 1980; 101(1):21–31.

17. Heidam HZ. Spontaneous abortion among dental assistants, factory workers, painters and gardening workers: a follow-up study. *J Epidemiol Community Health* 1984;38:149–155.
18. Rowland AS, Baird DD, Shore DL, et al. Nitrous oxide and spontaneous abortion in female dental assistants. *Am J Epidemiol* 1995;141:531–538.
19. Axelesson G, Ahlborg G Jr, Bodin L. Shift work, nitrous oxide exposure and spontaneous abortion among Swedish midwives. *Occup Environ Med* 1996;53:374–378.

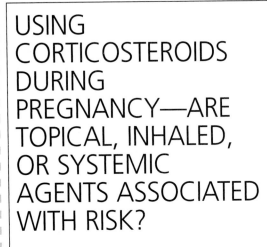

USING CORTICOSTEROIDS DURING PREGNANCY—ARE TOPICAL, INHALED, OR SYSTEMIC AGENTS ASSOCIATED WITH RISK?

Irena Nulman, MD
Shinya Ito, MD
Gideon Koren, MD, FRCPC

QUESTION

I am concerned about use of corticosteroids during pregnancy. Some of my women patients of reproductive age are using topical, inhaled, or oral preparations, and I am not sure what to advise.

Answer

Both topical and systemic corticosteroids are used for a variety of autoimmune and inflammatory conditions. Results of first-trimester studies were inconclusive and underpowered. Recent meta-analyses suggest a small but significant association between use of systemic corticosteroids during the first trimester and oral clefts. This is consistent with results of animal studies. No similar evidence exists for topical or inhaled corticosteroids, probably because of much lower systemic exposure.

Corticosteroids are used to treat a variety of conditions; discontinuing them during pregnancy sometime exacerbates these conditions. Corticosteroids are available alone or in combination with other drugs for systemic, inhaled, and topical use. Systemic corticosteroids are used for autoimmune and inflammatory conditions. Inhaled steroids are now first-line treatment for asthma. Topical corticosteroids are frequently used to treat allergic and inflammatory dermatologic diseases, such as atopic dermatitis and psoriasis. Existing data on the safety of corticosteroids during pregnancy, particularly during the first trimester, are often conflicting and difficult to interpret.

SYSTEMIC CORTICOSTEROIDS

Commonly used systemic corticosteroids include prednisone, cortisone, and the active metabolites of prednisone and dexamethasone. Corticosteroids cross human placenta[1]; fluorinated corticosteroids penetrate the placenta more rapidly.[2] The increased incidence of low birth weight and stillbirths reported in fetuses exposed to corticosteroids can often be linked to the conditions for which the mothers were given the drugs.[3]

Several studies have suggested an association between oral clefts and use of systemic corticosteroids,[4-6] but one case-control and several prospective cohort studies failed to show such an association.[7-12] A meta-analysis conducted by the Motherisk Program of 123,175 women who received oral corticosteroids during the first trimester showed a slightly increased risk of oral clefts. Pooled results of odds ratios (ORs) in case-control studies showed a three-fold increase in oral clefts among offsprings of women who received oral corticosteroids during pregnancy. When results of six cohort studies were pooled, no significant increase in oral clefts was seen. When the largest study (50,282 patients) was excluded because it did not distinguish between major and minor malformations, however, the OR increased to 3.03 (95% confidence interval 1.08 to 8.54) for major malformations in children whose mothers received corticosteroids during the first trimester of pregnancy.[3]

A recent prospective, controlled study followed 311 women who used various corticosteroids during the first trimester. Both corticosteroid-exposed women and controls had malformation rates within the expected baseline risk for the general population. The authors also recalculated a cumulative OR from seven controlled studies, including their own study, and found no significant increase in risk of major anomalies.[13]

Because most human studies of systemic corticosteroid use during pregnancy have looked at the drugs in combination with other medications, it is difficult to assess the risk of individual corticosteroids.

While systemic corticosteroids do not seem to pose a major teratogenic risk for humans, there is a small but significantly increased risk
of oral clefts with first-trimester exposure. These results are consistent with results of extensive studies in animals.[14,15]

INHALED CORTICOSTEROIDS

Inhaled corticosteroids used to treat asthma or other respiratory symptoms include beclomethasone, budesonide, flunisolide, fluticasone,
mometasone, and triamcinolone.[16]

It is estimated that up to 4% of all pregnancies are complicated by
maternal asthma,[17] making asthma one of the most common respiratory
complications seen in pregnancy. Poor control of chronic asthma and
exacerbation of acute asthma during pregnancy can result in adverse
maternal and fetal outcomes, such as hypoxia, low birth weight, and
intrauterine growth restriction.[18–20] A randomized controlled study has
shown that long-term use of low-dose budesonide decreases the risk of
severe exacerbations and improves asthma control in patients with mild,
persistent asthma of recent onset.[19] Inhaled steroids have also been
shown to reduce risk of hospitalization due to asthma.[21,22]

Epidemiologic data on inhaled corticosteroids have shown no
increase in rates of congenital malformations. A retrospective study of
women treated with triamcinolone, beclomethasone, and oral theo-
phylline for asthma during pregnancy found no congenital abnormalities in any treatment groups.[23] In addition, START (Inhaled Steroid
Treatment As Regular Therapy), the first long-term, multicentre,
prospective, double-blind study, reported that treating asthmatic pregnant women with 400 μg of budesonide is safe.[24]

These results corroborate data from the Swedish Registry Study[25]
of about 3000 pregnancies, which showed a normal rate of malformations in newborns exposed to budesonide during the first trimester.

Inhaled corticosteroids are currently recommended as part of routine
management of moderate-to-severe chronic asthma during pregnancy.[26]

TOPICAL CORTICOSTEROIDS

Commonly used topical corticosteroids include hydrocortisone and
betamethasone. The systemic effects of topical corticosteroids are
generally limited because only about 3% of the medication in topical

preparations is absorbed systemically following 8 hours of contact with normal skin.[27] Absorption varies with different types and doses of preparations and the nature and extent of underlying skin conditions. When corticosteroids are used long term or on large areas of skin, they might have systemic effects.[28-34]

Epidemiologic fetal safety data on topical corticosteroids are sparse. Two population-based studies found that treatment with topical corticosteroids during pregnancy did not increase risk of congenital abnormalities in humans.[35,36]

DISCUSSION

The apparent increased risk of oral clefts associated with systemic corticosteroid use has to be balanced against potentially serious implications for mothers (and indirectly fetuses) if needed steroid therapy is discontinued or not initiated for underlying maternal conditions. Since oral clefts occur at about one per thousand births, this increased risk will have a minimal absolute effect on the overall malformation rate of 3%. Since palate formation is completed by 12 weeks' gestation, no risk of oral clefts exists thereafter.

When exposure has already occurred, a level II ultrasound scan might be able to detect clefting. More studies are needed to determine which cleft phenotype is associated with corticosteroids and whether it is cleft lip (with or without palate) or cleft palate alone, or both.

REFERENCES

1. Briggs GG, Freeman RK, Yaffe SJ. Drugs in pregnancy and lactation: a reference guide to fetal and neonatal risk. 6th ed. Philadelphia, Pa: Lippincott Williams and Wilkins; 2002:662-670.
2. Mok CC, Wong RW. Pregnancy in systemic lupus erythematosus. *Postgrad Med J* 2001;77:157-165.
3. Park-Wyllie L, Mazzotta P, Pastuszak A, et al. Birth defects after maternal exposure to corticosteroids: prospective cohort study and meta-analysis of epidemiological studies. *Teratology* 2000;62:385-392.
4. Rodriguez-Pinilla E, Martinez-Frias ML. Corticosteroids during pregnancy and oral clefts: a case-control study. *Teratology* 1998;58:2-5.
5. Robert E, Vollset SE, Botto L, et al. Malformation surveillance and maternal drug exposure: the MADRE project. Int J Risk Safety Med 1994;6:78-118.
6. Carmichael SL, Shaw GM. Maternal corticosteroid use and risk of selected congenital anomalies. *Am J Med Genet* 1999;86:242-244.

7. Vickers CF. Double-blind trial of betamethasone. *BMJ* 1962;20: 156–157.

8. Warrell DW, Taylor R. Outcome for the foetus of mothers receiving prednisolone during pregnancy. *Lancet* 1968;1:117–118.

9. Heinonen OP, Slone D, Shapiro S. Antimicrobial and antiparasitic agents. *Birth Defects and Drugs in Pregnancy*. Littleton, Ma.: Publishing Sciences Group; 1977. p. 296–313.

10. Mogadam M, Dobbins WO, Korelitz BI, et al. Pregnancy in inflamatory bowel disease: effect of sulfasalazine and corticosteroid on fetal outcome. *Gastroenterology* 1981;80:72–76.

11. Mintz G, Niz J, Gutierrez G, et al. Prospective study of pregnancy in systemic lupus erythematosus. Results of a multidisciplinary approach. *J Rheumatol* 1986;13:732–739.

12. Czeizel AE, Rockenbauer M. Population-based case-control study of teratogenic potential of corticosteroids. *Teratology* 1997;56:355–340.

13. Gur C, Diav-Citrin O, Shechtman S, et al. Pregnancy outcome after first trimester exposure to corticosteroids: a prospective controlled study. *Reprod Toxicol* 2004;18:93–101.

14. Walker BE. Induction of cleft palate in rats with antiinflammatory drugs. *Teratology* 1971;4(1):39–42.

15. Pinsky L, Digeorge AM. Cleft palate in the mouse: a teratogenic index of glucocorticoid potency. *Science* 1965;147:402–403.

16. Passalacqua G, Albasno M, Canonica GW, et al. Inhaled and nasal corticosteroids: safety aspects. *Allergy* 2000;55:16–33.

17. Venkataraman MT, Shanies HM. Pregnancy and asthma. *J Asthma* 1997;34:265–271.

18. Witlin AG. Asthma in pregnancy. *Semin Perinatol* 1997;21:284–297.

19. Dombrowski MP. Pharmacologic therapy of asthma during pregnancy. *Obstet Gynecol Clin* North Am 1997;24:559–574.

20. Jana N, Vasishta K, Saha SC, et al. Effect of bronchial asthma on the course of pregnancy, labour and perinatal outcome. *J Obstet Gynaecol* 1995;21:227–232.

21. Pauwels RA, Pedersen S, Busse WW, et al. START Investigators Group. Early intervention with budesonide in mild persistent asthma: a randomised, double-blind trial. *Lancet* 2003;361:1071–1076.

22. Donahue JG, Weiss ST, Livingston JM, et al. Inhaled steroids and the risk of hospitalization for asthma. *JAMA* 1997;227:887–891.

23. Blais L, Suissa S, Boivin JF, et al. First treatment with inhaled corticosteroids and the prevention of admissions to hospital for asthma. *Thorax* 1998;53:1025–1029.

24. Silverman M, Sheffer A, Diaz Amor P, et al. Prospective pregnancy outcome data from the START study. On behalf of the safety committee. *Eur Respir J* 2002;20(Suppl 38):53S.

25. Norjavaara E, De Verdier MG. Normal pregnancy outcomes in a population-based study including 2,968 pregnant women exposed to budesonide. *J Allergy Clin Immunol* 2003;111:736–742.

26. Sheffer AL, Taggart VS, National Asthma Education Program. Expert panel report guidelines for the diagnosis and management of asthma.

National Heart, Lung, and Blood Institute. *Med Care* 1993;31(Suppl. 3): S20–S28.

27. Tauscher AE, Fleischer AB Jr, Phelps KC, et al. Psoriasis and pregnancy. *J Cutan Med Surg* 2002;6:561–570.

28. Hardman JG, Limbird LE, Gilman AG. Goodman & Gilman's *The Pharmacologic Basis of Therapeutics*. 7th ed. New York, NY: McGraw-Hill Medical Publishing Division; 1985. p. 1473.

29. Mizuchi A, Miyachi Y, Tamaki K, et al. Percutaneous absorption of betamethasone 17-benzoate measured by radioimmunoassay. *J Invest Dermatol* 1976;67:279–282.

30. Schaefer H, Zesch A, Stuttgen G. Penetration, permeation, and absorption of triamcinolone acetonide in normal and psoriatic skin. *Arch Dermatol Res* 1977;258:241–249.

31. Wester RC, Noonan PK, Maibach HI. Percutaneous absorption of hydrocortisone increases with long-term administration. In vivo studies in the rhesus monkey. *Arch Dermatol* 1980;116:186–188.

32. Turpeinen M. Absorption of hydrocortisone from the skin reservoir in atopic dermatitis. *Br J Dermatol* 1991;124:358–360.

33. Barnetson RS, White AD. The use of corticosteroids in dermatological practice. *Med J Aust* 1992;156:428–431.

34. Melendres JL, Bucks DA, Camel E, et al. In vivo percutaneous absorption of hydrocortisone: multiple-application dosing in man. *Pharm Res* 1992; 9:1164–1167.

35. Czeizel AE, Rockenbauer M. Population-based case-control study of teratogenic potential of corticosteroids. *Teratology* 1997;56:335–340.

36. Mygind H, Thulstrup AM, Pedersen L, et al. Risk of intrauterine growth retardation, malformations and other birth outcomes in children after topical use of corticosteroid in pregnancy. *Acta Obstet Gynecol Scand* 2002;81(3):234–239.

CHAPTER 29

NONSTEROIDAL ANTI-INFLAMMATORY DRUGS FOR RHEUMATOID ARTHRITIS DURING PREGNANCY

Gideon Koren, MD, FRCPC

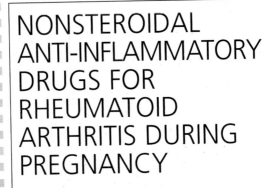

QUESTION

I am treating two pregnant patients who have rheumatoid arthritis (RA) with nonsteroidal anti-inflammatory drugs (NSAIDs). Are these medications safe at high doses during pregnancy?

Answer

While these medications do not appear to increase overall rates of congenital malformations, they do increase the risk of ductus arteriosus constriction or closure.

RA is a systemic autoimmune inflammatory disease of the joints. It affects women of reproductive age, so pregnancy complicated by RA is not uncommon. Most pregnant women find that RA tends to improve during pregnancy; it often improves during the second and third trimesters.

Treating RA during pregnancy is particularly challenging. NSAIDs are the mainstay of therapy, despite reported and confirmed adverse effects on both mothers and fetuses when they are used for long periods. The principal mode of action of this class of anti-inflammatory drugs is their nonselective inhibition of cyclooxygenases 1 and 2 (COX-1 and COX-2). In addition to the desired effect of reducing inflammation, non-selective COX inhibitors also inhibit gastric, platelet, and renal production of prostaglandin.[1]

All NSAIDs cross the human placenta and are distributed to the fetus at term. Prenatal exposure to NSAIDs has been shown to increase the incidence of pulmonary hypertension, premature closure of the ductus arteriosus, and periventricular hemorrhage, and to impair fetal renal function leading to oligohydramnios.[2] These effects have been reported for indomethacin, ibuprofen, ketoprofen, and diclofenac.[1] Although risk of ductal closure increases during late pregnancy in women exposed to NSAIDs, closure is frequently resolved within 24 hours of stopping therapy.

Fetuses exposed to NSAIDs often have decreased urinary output,[1] but as with ductal closure, the amniotic fluid usually returns to normal after therapy is stopped. Renal complications appear to be rare, considering the number of women treated with NSAIDs.[3] Adverse renal effects reported include fatal anuria, renal failure, oliguria, and oligohydramnios.

A population-based retrospective study on use of NSAIDs showed that they did not increase adverse birth outcomes, but did increase risk of miscarriage.[4] Although the sample size was large with no apparent selection bias, the study's retrospective design limits the reliability of its results.

Ostensen and Ostensen[1] prospectively studied pregnant women with rheumatic disease to compare the incidence of adverse fetal effects between women exposed and not exposed to NSAIDs. They found no increased risk of teratogenicity or neonatal adverse outcomes in the group exposed to NSAIDs. Fetal echocardiographic studies were not conducted, however, so risk of transient ductal closure and reduced amniotic fluid volume could not be evaluated.

The only two NSAIDs extensively studied in pregnant women are acetylsalicylic acid (ASA) and indomethacin. The Motherisk team recently reviewed ASA therapy[5] and concluded that, overall, there was no increased risk of congenital malformations among fetuses exposed to ASA in utero. Case-control studies, however, showed an association between ASA and the rare condition gastroschisis. In most of these studies, ASA was used for upper respiratory tract infections, so it is possible that gastroschisis was induced by respiratory viruses. This possibility is attractive because gastroschisis has been associated also with a different drug used for upper respiratory tract infections, n-propanalamine.

Indomethacin has been linked to a variety of adverse fetal effects, documented in several trials.[6–9] One study,[6] found an increased incidence of pulmonary hypertension in the indomethacin group. Eronen et al.[9]

also found an increased incidence of respiratory distress syndrome, bronchopulmonary dysplasia, and necrotizing enterocolitis in their indomethacin-exposed group.

A recent meta-analysis completed by Motherisk[10] found a 15-fold increased risk of ductal constriction after brief (up to 48 hours) exposure to NSAIDs near term. No such risk seems to exist with use of NSAIDs during the first two trimesters. These data suggest a cautious approach, as it is likely that chronic use of NSAIDs in high doses, such as is necessary in the treatment of RA, is associated with an increased risk of adverse fetal effects.

REFERENCES

1. Ostensen M, Ostensen H. Safety of nonsteroidal antiinflammatory drugs in pregnant patients with rheumatic disease. *J Rheumatol* 1996;23(6): 1045–1049.
2. Hernández-Díaz S, García-Rodríguez LA. Epidemiologic assessment of the safety of conventional nonsteroidal anti-inflammatory drugs. *Am J Med* 2001;110 (3 check globally Suppl. 1):20S–27S.
3. Cuzzolin L, Dal Cere M, Fanos V. NSAID-induced nephrotoxicity from the fetus to the child. *Drug Saf* 2001;24(1):9–18.
4. Nielsen GL, Sorensen HT, Larsen H, et al. Risk of adverse birth outcome and miscarriage in pregnant users of non-steroidal anti-inflammatory drugs: population based observational study and case-control study. *BMJ* 2001;322(7281):266–270.
5. Kozer E, Costei AM, Boskovic R, et al. Effects of aspirin consumption during pregnancy on pregnancy outcomes: meta-analysis. *Birth Defects Res B Dev Reprod Toxicol* 2003;68(1):70–84.
6. Besinger RE, Niebyl JR, Keyes WG, et al. Randomized comparative trial of indomethacin and ritodrine for the long-term treatment of preterm labor. *Am J Obstet Gynecol* 1991;164(4):981–986. Discussion. *Am J Obstet Gynecol* 1991;164(4):986–988.
7. Kurki T, Eronen M, Lumme R, et al. A randomized double-dummy comparison between indomethacin and nylidrin in threatened preterm labor. *Obstet Gynecol* 1991;78(6):1093–1097.
8. Morales WJ, Smith SG, Angel JL, et al. Efficacy and safety of indomethacin versus ritodrine in the management of preterm labor: a randomized study. *Obstet Gynecol* 1989;74(4):567–572.
9. Eronen M, Pesonen E, Kurki T, et al. Increased incidence of bronchopulmonary dysplasia after antenatal administration of indomethacin to prevent preterm labor. *J Pediatr* 1994;124(5 Pt. 1):782–788.
10. Costei AM, Florescu A, Boskovic R, et al. NSAIDs during the third trimester and the risk of premature closure of the ductus arteriosus: a meta-analysis. In press.

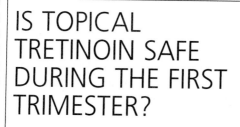

CHAPTER 30

IS TOPICAL TRETINOIN SAFE DURING THE FIRST TRIMESTER?

Gideon Koren, MD, FRCPC

QUESTION

One of my patients conceived while using a topical tretinoin preparation for acne. I know this drug is related to Accutane, which is teratogenic. How should I advise her?

Answer

Available evidence suggests that topical tretinoin does not increase teratogenic risk in humans.

The first-generation retinoid, *cis*-retinoic acid (CRA, isotretinoin) is derived from the endogenous isomerization of all-*trans* retinoic acid (TRA), which is derived from diet and retinol metabolites. Both CRA and TRA, endogenous constituents of serum, are essential for vision, reproduction, metabolism, differentiation, and the spatial organization of cells within a developing organ.[1]

TRA is marketed as a topical tretinoin preparation (Retin-A, Renova) for treatment of acne vulgaris and photodamage. *Cis*-retinoic acid is marketed as the oral isotretinoin preparation, Accutane. Isotretinoin is a confirmed human teratogen, and its use is contraindicated during pregnancy due to the serious risk of physical and developmental anomalies that could result from first-trimester exposure.[2,3]

Studies have described a retinoid embryopathy consisting of craniofacial, cardiac, thymic, and central nervous system abnormalities.[3] It is thought that the metabolic activation of isotretinoin to TRA might be responsible for its teratogenicity.[4]

Oral tretinoin has produced dose- and stage-dependent fetal anomalies in several animal models.[5-7] No teratogenic effects have been reported in pregnant women, but, according to the *United States Pharmacopoeia Dispensing Information*,[8] topical tretinoin should not be used during pregnancy.

Published information on pregnancy outcome following maternal exposure to topical tretinoin is limited to two case reports, three epidemiologic studies, voluntary reports submitted to the U.S. Food and Drug Administration, and articles from the company that makes the product.[9-14]

With growing interest in using topical tretinoin products to combat changes to the skin from aging, the population of users will expand from teenagers using it to treat acne to young and middle-aged adults. This new group of individuals clearly includes women in their childbearing years. Use of topical tretinoin on a long-term basis has prompted concern about the possibility of increased circulating concentrations of tretinoin and its metabolites.[15] Given the paucity of prospectively controlled collected data, we recently compared the rate of major malformations in fetuses of women exposed to tretinoin (all of whom were counseled by Motherisk while pregnant) with the rate in fetuses of women not exposed.[16]

We were able to ascertain pregnancy outcome for 94 of the 131 (72%) women in the cohort. All patients reported first-trimester exposure. Only a few could remember continuing the medication beyond the first trimester, and none used it to term. Patients reported exposure to a range of tretinoin preparations; 17% of patients could not recall the strength of preparation they had used. All patients applied tretinoin to their faces. Most were treating acne vulgaris; one patient used the medication for photodamage. No patient was exposed to isotretinoin. Most patients were taking prenatal multivitamins containing 1500 IU of vitamin A. Tretinoin-exposed patients and their controls were similar in many respects (Table 30-1). The women exposed to tretinoin were more likely to be primigravidas (55/94 vs. 53/133, $P = 0.008$).

We lacked information on pregnancy outcome for 37 of the 131 women in the study cohort. Of these 37, 24 could not be contacted at the telephone number they had given at the Motherisk intake call, 3 had given a workplace number but were away on maternity leave and the workplace would not divulge a home number, and 10 were

TABLE 30-1
MOTHERS' CHARACTERISTICS

Characteristic	Mothers Exposed To Tretinoin (N = 94)	Controls (N = 133)	P Value
Age (years)*	30.4 ± 4.7	31.2 ± 4.7	0.25
Nonsmokers	84 (89%)	124 (93%)	0.29
Alcohol consumers† • Abstainers • Heavy drinkers	71 (76%) 8 (9%)	102 (77%) 6 (5%)	0.97 0.34
Gravidity • G1 • ≥ G2	55 (59%) 39 (41%)	53 (40%) 80 (60%)	0.008 0.008
Parity • P0 • P1 • P2 • P3 • ≥ P4	62 (66%) 21 (22%) 9 (10%) 1 (1%) 0	7 (5%) 69 (52%) 40 (30%) 10 (8%) 7 (5%)	0.001 0.001 0.005 0.06 0.06
Miscarriages • S0 • S1 • S2 • ≥ S3	87 (93%) 7 (7%) 0 0	96 (72%) 28 (21%) 5 (4%) 3 (2%)	0.001 0.01 0.15 0.38
No elective abortionsÜ	86 (91%)	113 (86%)	0.20
Prepregnancy weight (kg)*	57.7	60.1	0.21

* Unpaired Student's *t* test.
† x^2 test.

physicians inquiring about their pregnant patients so insufficient data were available for follow-up.

Ninety-four women gave birth to 86 live infants, including 1 set of twins. Pregnancy outcome was similar among controls (Table 30-2). There was no statistical difference in rates of live births, miscarriages, or elective terminations. There were no perinatal deaths.

TABLE 30-2
PREGNANCY OUTCOME

Pregnancy Outcome	Mothers Exposed To Tretinoin	Controls	P Value
Live births	86*/94 (91%)	119/133 (89%)	0.99
Miscarriage	6/94	12/133	0.63
Elective termination	3/94	2/133	0.69
Major malformations in live births	2/86 (2%)	4/119 (3%)	0.30†
Gestational age (wk)	39.6 ± 1.5 (range 35 to 42)	39.6 ± 1.5 (range 36 to 42)	0.99
Premature (<37 wk)	4/86 (5%)	5/119 (4%)	0.25†
Birth weight (g)	3354.5 ± 470.2 (range 2272 to 4487)	3501.9 ± 553.5 (range 2074 to 5396)	0.05
Low birth weight (<2500 g)	4/84 (5%)	4/119 (3%)	0.25†
Caesarean section	19/86 (22%)	24/119 (20%)	0.81
Vaginal delivery	67/86 (78%)	95/119 (80%)	

* Includes a set of twins.

† Fisher's exact test.

The incidence of major malformations among live-born babies exposed to tretinoin during the first trimester did not differ between groups (Table 30-2). The major defects in tretinoin-exposed infants were bicuspid aortic valves and dysplastic kidneys. Neither of these defects are consistent with known retinoic acid embryopathy. Defects among controls were two congenitally dislocated hips, one aortic valvular stenosis, and one imperforate anus.

No difference between groups was noticed for method of delivery, gestational age, or preterm delivery (Table 30-2). Babies in the control group had a mean birth weight 148 g heavier than babies in the study group. After removing one large control infant (5396 g), however, the difference was not statistically significant. Poststudy analysis did not reveal a relationship between tretinoin concentration and birth weight.

Acne vulgaris is common among women of childbearing age. Symptomatic treatment with topical tretinoin is common. Tretinoin is also used to treat photodamage. Since 50% of pregnancies are unplanned, and women are delaying pregnancy until later in life, women might well become pregnant while using tretinoin.

Our study includes the largest sample to date of women known to have used topical tretinoin during early pregnancy. Results failed to show increased risk of congenital malformations among these women. The two infants in the exposed group who were born with major malformations did not have the phenotype of retinoid embryopathy.

No relationship was found between drug exposure and method of delivery, gestational age, or preterm delivery. The difference in birth weight between the two groups is likely explained by one infant born at 41 weeks weighing 5396 g.

A potential limitation of our study was its inability to detect a smaller than sixfold increase in the risk of malformations. Both study and control groups, however, had major malformation rates well within parameters expected, and no infant had a retinoid-type embryopathy.

While we need additional information on the concentration of retinoids in embryos with various exposures, these concentrations are unlikely to be above endogenous levels.[15,17–23] This study helps put in context the warnings in the various product monographs that caution against tretinoin use during pregnancy.

REFERENCES

1. Goodman D. Vitamin A and retinoids in health and disease. N Engl J Med 1984;310:1023–1031.
2. De la Cruz E, Sun S, Vangvanichyakorn K. Multiple congenital malformations associated with maternal isotretinoin therapy. Pediatrics 1984;74: 428–430.
3. Lammer E, Chen D, Hoar R, et al. Retinoic acid embryopathy. N Engl J Med 1985;313:837–841.
4. Creech KJ, Lammer E, Olney A. Embryonic retinoid concentrations after maternal intake of isotretinoin. N Engl J Med 1989;321:262.
5. Kistler A. Teratogenesis of retinoic acid in rats: susceptible stages and suppression of retinoic acid-induced limb malformations by cycloheximide. Teratology 1981;23:25–31.
6. Kochhar DM. Teratogenic activity of retinoic acid. Acta Pathol Microbiol Scand 1967;70:398–404.

7. Seegmiller RE, Ford WH, Carter MW, et al. A developmental toxicity study of tretinoin administered topically and orally to pregnant Wistar rats. *J Am Acad Dermatol* 1997;36(Suppl.):S60–S66.

8. United States Pharmacopoeial Convention. *United States Pharmacopoeia Dispensing Information*. Rockville, MD: US Pharmacopoeia Convention; 1997.

9. Reed B. Pregnancy, drugs and the dermatologist. *Curr Probl Dermatol* 1994;6:72–80.

10. Rosa F. Holoprosencephaly with first trimester topical tretinoin. *Teratology* 1994;49:418.

11. Camera G, Pregliasco P. Ear malformation in baby born to mother using tretinoin cream. *Lancet* 1992;339:687.

12. Lipson A, Collins F, Webster W. Multiple congenital defects associated with maternal use of topical tretinoin. *Lancet* 1993;341:1352–1353.

13. Jick SS, Terris BZ, Jick H. First trimester topical tretinoin and congenital disorders. *Lancet* 1993;341:1181–1182.

14. DeWals P, Bloch D, Calabro A, et al. Association between holoprosen-cephaly and exposure to topical retinoids: results of the EUROCAT survey. *Pediatr Perinatol Epidemiol* 1991;5:445–447.

15. Johnson K, Chambers C, Felix R, et al. Pregnancy outcome in women prospectively ascertained with retin-A exposures: an ongoing study. *Teratol Soc Abst* 1994:375.

16. Shapiro L, Pastuszak A, Curto G, et al. Safety of first trimester exposure to topical tretinoin. *Lancet* 1997;350:1134–4.

17. Latriano L, Tzimas G, Wong F, et al. The percutaneous absorption of top-ically applied tretinoin and its effect on endogenous concentrations of tretinoin and its metabolites after single doses or long-term use. *J Am Acad Dermatol* 1997;36(Suppl):S37–S46.

18. Schaefer H, Zesch A. Penetration of vitamin A into human skin. *Acta Derm Venerol* (Stockh) 1975;74:50–55.

19. Chiang T-C. Gas chromatographic-mass spectrometric assay for low lev-els of retinoic acid in human blood. *J Chromatogr* 1980;182:335–340.

20. Franz T, Lehman P. Systemic absorption of retinoic acid. *J Toxicol Cutan Ocular Toxicol* 1989;8:517–524.

21. Franz T, Lehman PA, Franz SF. Topical use of retinoic acid gel is not ter-atogenic. *J Invest Dermatol* 1993;100:490.

22. Buchan P. Evaluation of the teratogenic risk of cutaneously administered retinoids. *Skin Pharmacol* 1993;(Suppl. 1):45–52.

23. Kemper C, Holland ML, Thorne EG. Percutaneous absorption of 3H-tretinoin following long-term administration of topical tretinoin. *Dermatologica* 1990;181:351.

CHAPTER 31

HOW TO ENSURE FETAL SAFETY WHEN MOTHERS USE ISOTRETINOIN (ACCUTANE)

Gideon Koren, MD, FRCPC

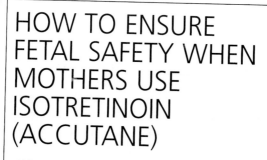

QUESTION

I have a female patient with acne who was prescribed Accutane by a dermatologist. She was told about the risk to the baby and was asked to sign some documents. Is this legal?

Answer

The Pregnancy Prevention Program (PPP) should be the standard of care for women of reproductive age using isotretinoin. Primary care physicians should be responsible for ensuring that women know the serious teratogenic risk of this product.

When thalidomide was demonstrated to be a potent human teratogen, it was immediately removed from the market. isotretinoin and etretinate were introduced to the market with full knowledge of their animal teratogenicity, which had been established in animal studies[1] Isotretinoin (13-*cis*-Retinoic acid; Accutane) is used to treat severe cystic acne that has proven recalcitrant to standard therapy; etretinate (Tegison) is prescribed for patients with psoriasis and other keratinization disorders. Both drugs currently are contraindicated in pregnancy.

Based on the half-lives of elimination, women discontinuing isotretinoin are advised not to conceive before 1 calendar month has elapsed. Those stopping etretinate are frequently advised that the safe time to wait before conceiving has not yet been established. In some cases, prescribing physicians suggest a waiting period of 2 to 3 years before patients should conceive.

Tragically enough, despite clear labeling of isotretinoin as contraindicated during pregnancy, birth defects consequent to in utero exposure were reported soon after its distribution.

The pattern of isotretinoin embryophaty is now well-known and includes serious craniofacial, central nervous system, cardiovascular, and thymic malformations. Ear abnormalities include microtia, low-set ears, and anotia; central nervous system defects include microcephalus, hydrocephalus, and reduction malformations of the brain. Cardiovascular defects include transposition of the great arteries, Fallot's tetralogy, ventral septal defects, and aortic arch abnormalities.[2]

Acknowledging that routine labeling of isotretinoin as teratogenic was not sufficient to prevent fetal exposure, the manufacturer and the Food and Drug Administration in the United States developed a PPP for isotretinoin, which consists of printed material for prescribing physicians to use in educating female patients about the serious risk for birth defects.[3] Etretinate has not been labeled as a serious human teratogen in the medical literature yet. However, because it is a synthetic retinoid and a derivative of vitamin A, like isotretinoin, doctors have exercised extreme caution when counseling women of reproductive age about conception during and after etretinate therapy.

The PPP, and unprecedented program, contains an information brochure for patients, a qualification checklist, and a line drawing of a hypothetical isotretinoin-exposed fetus. Female patients are asked to sign a consent form acknowledging that they have been instructed through the PPP, that they are aware of the need to use contraception during isotretinoin therapy, and that they will undergo pregnancy testing before, during and after isotretinoin therapy. The PPP stresses and suggests simultaneous use of two forms of contraception in an attempt to further reduce the likelihood of fetal exposure. The PPP for isotretinoin was distributed to all isotretinoin-prescribing physicians in Canada in October 1988, and a similar PPP for etretinate followed in 1989. Despite this campaign to better inform women about the teratogenic risks of retinoids, fetal exposure to these drugs still occurs. Special attention must be paid to the factors that lead to fetal exposure, because any strategy that aims to reduce fetal exposure must begin with an understanding of the mechanisms that lead to it.

We prospectively analyzed a group of isotretinoin- and etretinate-exposed women who contacted the Motherisk Program for counseling about reproductive risks.[4] Using a standardized questionnaire, we

TABLE 31-1

Characteristic	Isotretinoin-Exposed Women N = 26	Matched controls N = 26	P Value
Mean age at first consultation (SD)	25.2 (±6.7)	28.9 (±5.1)	0.03
Number of adolescents (≤ 20 y)	9	1	0.014
Marital status • Single • Married • Data not available	11 12 3	8 18 	NS
Ethnic background • White • Black • Oriental • Persian • East Indian • Data not available	22 3 1 0 0 0	18 0 1 1 2 4	NS
Mean gestational age (wk) at first consultation (SD)	10.2 (±8)	6 (±4.2)	0.01
Referal to Motherisk • Physician • Self	20 6	21 5	NS
Number of alcoholic drinks per day • 0 • ≤ 1 • 1–2 • Data not available	15 6 0 5	17 7 0 0	NS
Mean number of cigarettes smoked per day by admitted smokers (SD)	1.3 (±4.4)	3.6 (±7.3)	NS
Mean socioeconomic index (0 = lowest, 100 = highest) (SD)	44.3 (±16.1)	43.9 (±23.6)	NS

TABLE 31-1 (Continued)

Characteristic	Isotretinoin-Exposed Women N = 26	Matched controls N = 26	P Value
Mean gravidity (SD)	1.7 (±1.5)	1.9 (±1.4)	NS
Mean parity (SD)	0.5 (±0.6)	0.6 (±0.7)	NS
Mean number of previous therapeuticabortions (SD)	0.1 (±0.4)	0.2 (±0.4)	NS
Mean number of previous spontaneous abortions (SD)	0.2 (±0.7)	0.4 (±0.7)	NS

investigated and reported maternal demographic characteristics, degree of use of the PPP, and pattern of contraception after they were seen by the physicians who prescribed the synthetic retinoids.

We included women who voluntarily contacted the Motherisk Program from November 1, 1988, to January 30, 1991, for counseling after exposure to systemic retinoids. Marital status, socioeconomic status, gravity, parity, previous miscarriages and elective abortions, maternal tobacco and ethanol exposure, contraception use, and use of the PPP (educational components, patient recollection of warnings) were recorded (Table 31-1).

The 26 isotretinoin-exposed women were younger than controls (next case attending the clinic) (25.2 [SD 6.7] years vs. 28.9 [SD 5.1] years, P = 0.03). tended to be adolescent (30.8% vs. 3.8%, P = 0.014), and sought counseling later in gestation (10.1 [SD 8] weeks vs. 6 [SD 4.2] weeks, P = 0.01). Of the 20 (77%) who knew the drug was teratogenic, 10 (38.5%) used no contraception, 6 (23.1%) experienced method failure, and 2 (8%) stopped contraception during isotretinoin therapy. Although cognizant of the teratogenicity of isotretinoin, more than one-third of the women in this study used no birth control or experienced contraception failure. In this same group, however compliance with contraception use appeared to increase in those with more exposure to the PPP.

REFERENCES

1. Kamm JJ. Toxicology, carcinogenicity and teratogenicity of some orally administered retinoids. *J Am Acad Dermatol* 1982;6:652–659.
2. Lammer EJ, Chen DT, Hoar RM, et al. Retinoic acid embryophathy. *N Engl J Med* 1985;313:387–341.
3. Pastuszak AL, Koren G. The Retinoid Pregnancy Prevention Program. In: Koren G. ed. *Retinoids in Clinical Practice. The risk-benefit ratio.* New York: Marcel Dekker, 1993:147–175.
4. Pastuszak AL, Koren G, Rieder M. Use of the retinoid pregnancy prevention program in Canada. *Reprod Toxicol* 1994;8:63–68.

CHAPTER 32

YOUNG WOMEN TAKING ISOTRETINOIN STILL CONCEIVE: ROLE OF PHYSICIANS IN PREVENTING DISASTER

Gideon Koren, MD, FRCPC

QUESTION

One of my adolescent patients was prescribed isotretinoin for severe acne by a dermatologist. I was shocked to discover she does not use any means of contraception. The dermatologist insists he told her about the need for contraception. How can we do better?

Answer

Clearly this dermatologist, like many of his colleagues, does not comply with the Pregnancy Prevention Program (PPP). Until physicians become more aware of this program, babies will continue to be born with embryopathy due to isotretinoin.

Isotretinoin was introduced for clinical use 16 years ago as effective treatment for severe cystic acne, and more than 100,000 female patients are exposed to isotretinoin yearly in the United States.[1] Because preclinical studies of laboratory animals showed isotretinoin to be teratogenic,[2] and because the elimination half-life was relatively short (14.7 hours) in healthy volunteers,[3] the drug was contraindicated for women who were or might become pregnant during therapy and in the month following discontinuation of therapy. It soon became apparent, however, that women conceived while receiving the medication, and rates of teratogenicity were high.

The patterns of retinoic acid embryopathy are well-known today. They include central nervous system, cardiovascular, craniofacial, and thymic malformations.[4] Cognitive deficits in more than half the children exposed in utero have also been reported in follow-up studies to 5 years of age.[5]

Because standard labeling of the medication was not shown to prevent fetal exposure to isotretinoin, a PPP for isotretinoin was developed by the manufacturer and the U.S. Food and Drug Administration. The program includes printed material for prescribing physicians to use in educating female patients about the serious risk for birth defects[6] and instructions for physicians to obtain negative pregnancy test results before prescribing the drug and to delay therapy until the second or third day of the next normal menstrual period. The program strongly suggests simultaneous use of two forms of contraception in an attempt to further reduce the likelihood of fetal exposure. In addition, female patients are asked to sign a consent form acknowledging that they have been instructed through the PPP, that they are aware of the need for contraception during isotretinoin therapy, and that they will undergo pregnancy testing before, during, and after isotretinoin therapy.[7,8]

Despite these precautions, the Motherisk Program's teratogen information service in Toronto still records new cases of fetal exposure to isotretinoin every year.[9] We recently published four new cases of isotretinoin exposure during pregnancy to highlight continuing problems in implementing the PPP because of patients' and physicians' noncompliance.[9]

CASE 1

A 17-year-old woman in her first pregnancy gave birth following exposure to 60 mg/day of isotretinoin from 3 months before conception to the end of her first trimester. Her physician verbally advised her that, while receiving therapy with this medication, she should not conceive and that, if she became sexually active, she should use contraception. She also received pamphlets on isotretinoin. Although she fully understood the meaning of the information provided, she chose not to use contraception because "she did not intend to have sex."

Her pregnancy was diagnosed at 23 weeks' gestation. She was informed about the option of terminating the pregnancy and was offered the telephone number of an appropriate clinic. She decided to continue the pregnancy. Level 2 ultrasound examination did not reveal any abnormalities.

A male infant of 3000 g was born after full-term pregnancy by normal vaginal delivery. The infant, who did not cry at birth, experienced neonatal respiratory distress. His Apgar score was 1/5 (1 minute/5 minute, respectively). His head was microcephalic (32cm, <3%), and his facial features included a cupped thickened helix, a depressed nasal bridge, a cleft of soft and hard palate (without family history), and micrognathia. On two-dimensional echocardiographic examination, a small patent ductus arteriosus was detected.

CASE 2

A 20-year-old woman in her second pregnancy took twenty 10-mg tablets of isotretinoin during the first 4 weeks of an unplanned pregnancy. The medication had been prescribed the previous year for cystic acne by a dermatologist, but she had not taken it at that time. The woman was informed verbally by her physician about the teratogenic effects of isotretinoin and advised about proper contraception. She was not informed about the PPP and did not receive any printed material. She reported using birth control pills, but not regularly.

Even though she was informed about the increased risk of having a baby with major malformations, she decided to continue the pregnancy. She did not know the date of her last menstrual period, and ultrasound examination at 17 weeks' gestation did not show fetal abnormalities. She delivered a full-term baby by cesarean section. At birth, apart from hydrocele, the infant appeared normal.

CASE 3

A 16-year-old adolescent was prescribed 40 mg of isotretinoin daily for cystic acne by her dermatologist. She was told she should not conceive while receiving therapy, and a blood test was done to exclude pregnancy before initiation of therapy. She did not receive the PPP or any other written material. She visited her family physician, who prescribed birth control pills. She started isotretinoin treatment before results from the pregnancy test were obtained. Results were positive. In the meantime, she had taken three isotretinoin tablets. Because she did not remember the date of her last period, ultrasound examination was performed to determine the exact time of exposure, which turned out to be at 9 weeks' gestation. She was counseled by her physician and she contacted the Motherisk Program regarding the risks associated with isotretinoin exposure. After counseling she decided to continue the pregnancy until ultrasound examination results were obtained.

Even though results were negative for major malformations at 18 weeks' gestation, she decided to terminate the pregnancy. Pathologic findings after termination revealed no obvious internal or external abnormalities.

CASE 4

A 21-year-old woman in her first pregnancy was treated for cystic acne with 40 mg of isotretinoin daily by her dermatologist. She was informed about the teratogenic effects of isotretinoin, received the PPP, and signed the consent form. For contraception she chose condoms. Six weeks after discontinuing the drug, she found out she was pregnant. Because she did not know the date of her last menstrual period, ultrasound examination was performed. It showed she had conceived around the date she discontinued therapy. She delivered a full-term baby by cesarean section. At birth the infant was healthy and had no evident malformations.

DISCUSSION

Half the pregnancies in North America are unplanned and might result in inadvertent fetal exposure to drugs.[10] In 1994, we documented the demographic characteristics and pattern of use of contraceptives of Canadian women prescribed synthetic retinoic acids whose contraceptive methods failed. Our data showed that isotretinoin-exposed women were younger than their nonexposed controls, tended to be adolescents, and sought counseling later in gestation. The PPP for isotretinoin was reasonably used by prescribing physicians in the first years, as documented by a trend to more appropriate use of contraception by patients counseled with the entire program.[7]

During the last 6 months, the Motherisk Program has recorded four new cases of isotretinoin exposure during pregnancy. All four patients were younger than 22 years, and all four pregnancies were unplanned. This might indicate that the potential risk was not considered seriously by this group. The three who used contraception used a single method (Table 32-1), which is not the intent of the program.

All the women were verbally advised by their dermatologists not to conceive while receiving therapy and, if they were sexually active, to use contraception. Only one, however was given the full PPP and signed the consent form. In case 3, the dermatologist did not follow the program guideline and did not wait until obtaining pregnancy test results, which led to starting isotretinoin after the patient was already pregnant.

It could be argued that these four cases do not necessarily reflect widespread physician noncompliance with the program. A recent letter from a Canadian dermatologist practicing in British Columbia, however, substantiates our suspicions that these cases stem from widespread noncompliance by dermatologists, who are supposed to be the only specialists prescribing isotretinoin in Canada.[11]

The best prevention program is doomed to fail if physicians do not adhere to it. Our cases indicate that full compliance is still an issue, as in case 4. Regulatory agencies, manufacturers, and especially prescribing physicians should ensure that fetal exposure to isotretinoin is prevented. Continuous failure to implement the PPP and, in particular, to ensure contraception strongly suggests that prescription of isotretinoin should be coupled with referral to professional contraception counseling. Very

TABLE 32-1
COMPLIANCE WITH THE PREGNANCY PREVENTION PROGRAM IN
THE FOUR CASES

Compliance	Case 1	Case 2	Case 3	Case 4
Patient acknowledges knowing of risk	Yes	Yes	Yes	Yes
Physician mentioned teratogenic risk	Yes	Yes	Yes	Yes
Pregnancy Prevention Program was introduced	No	No	No	Yes
Using two modes of contraception simultaneously was mentioned	No	No	No	No
Patient signed consent form	No	No	No	Yes
Contraception was used	No*	Yes†	Yes‡	Yes§

* Patient did not intend to be sexually active.

† Used oral contraceptives but irregularly.

‡ Oral contraceptives were started before isotretinoin, but woman was already pregnant, as was later confirmed by blood test.

§ Condoms were used.

often, young teenagers have little sexual experience and poor understanding of birth control methods, which substantially increases the risk
of fetal exposure to isotretinoin.[8] In addition, an educational program for
physicians is needed to heighten awareness of this serious problem.

REFERENCES

1. Dai WS, La Braico JM, Stern RS. Epidemiology of isotretinoin exposure during pregnancy. *J Am Acad Dermatol* 1992;26:599–606.
2. Kochhar DM. Teratogenic activity of retinoic acid. *Acta Pathol Microbiol Scand* 1967;70:398–404.
3. Colburn WA, Gibson DM. Isotretinoin kinetics after 80 to 320 mg oral doses. *Clin Pharmacol Ther* 1985;37:411–414.
4. Lammer EJ, Chen DT, Hoar RM, et al. Retinoic acid embryopathy. *N Engl J Med* 1985;313:837–841.

5. Teratology Society. Recommendations for isotretinoin use in women of childbearing potential. *Teratology* 1991;44:1–6.

6. Pastuszak AL, Koren G. The Retinoid Pregnancy Prevention Program. In: Koren G, ed. *Retinoids in clinical practice. The risk-benefit ratio.* New York, NY: Marcel Dekker; 1993:147–175.

7. Pastuszak AL, Koren G, Rieder JM. Use of the retinoid pregnancy prevention program in Canada: patterns of contraception use in women treated with isotretinoin and etretinate. *Res Toxicol* 1994;8:63–68.

8. Koren G, Feldman Y, Shear N. Motherisk: a new approach to antenatal counseling of drug/chemical exposure. *Vet Hum Toxicol* 1986;28: 563–565.

9. Atanackovic G, Koren G. Failure of the Pregnancy Prevention Program for isotretinoin: analysis of recent Canadian cases. *Can Med Assoc J.* In press.

10. Skrabanek P. Smoking and statistical overkill. *Lancet* 1992;340:1208–1209.

11. Gregory WB. Isotretinoin and teratogenicity [letter]. *Can J Clin Pharmacol* 1997;4(3):3.

HYPOTHYROIDISM DURING PREGNANCY

Alejandro A. Nava-Ocampo, MD
Gideon Koren, MD, FRCPC

QUESTION

I have a 27-year-old patient diagnosed with hypothyroidism in the 8th week of pregnancy. She received conflicting opinions regarding risk for her baby and wants to get more information. I also found conflicting information in the literature. How should I advise her?

Answer

Pregnant patients with untreated hypothyroidism are at increased risk of obstetric complications. Adequate treatment with thyroid hormones greatly reduces the frequency of these complications. Observational studies suggest that children whose mothers had hypothyroxinemia in early pregnancy have lower IQs than matched controls. Another study has shown that even if levothyroxine therapy is started after the first trimester, there is an excellent chance children will have normal neuropsychologic development.

Hypothyroidism occurs during pregnancy relatively frequently. A nationwide U.S. survey showed that 4.6% of the population 12 years old and older had hypothyroidism and that 4.3% of all women suffered from thyroid disease or goitre, or were taking thyroid medication.[1] Routine prenatal screening showed that 2.2% of pregnant women in their second trimester had thyroid-stimulating hormone (TSH) levels at or above 6 mU/L.[2] Pregnant patients with hypothyroidism are at increased risk of obstetric complications, such as fetal death, gestational hypertension, placental abruption, and poor perinatal outcome. Adequate treatment with thyroid hormones greatly reduces the frequency of these maternal complications.[3]

Until 12 weeks' gestation, before the fetal thyroid begins to produce thyroid hormones, the developing brain is critically dependent on circulating levels of maternal thyroxine (T_4).[4] A recent trial demonstrated that thyroid insufficiency in pregnant rats disrupted migration of neurons in the fetal cortex and hippocampus, leading to aberrant location of neurons in the adult offspring's brain.[5] Children born to women with high serum TSH concentrations at 17 weeks' gestation who were not treated for hypothyroidism had 7-point lower IQs than matched controls.[6] A prospective cohort study has shown that low levels of free thyroxine (fT_4) at 12 weeks' gestation are associated with impaired psychomotor development at 10 months old.[7]

TREATMENT

Two thyroid hormones, levothyroxine (L-T_4) and liothyronine (L-T_3), are available in Canada. L-T_3 can be used occasionally when quick onset of action is required, but is less desirable for chronic replacement therapy because it requires frequent dosing and because it produces a transient elevation in triiodothyronine concentrations.

A desiccated hormone preparation, derived from animal thyroids, is also available in Canada. It contains both thyroxine and triiodothyronine, but because it has highly variable biologic activity, it is not recommended as the primary alternative for thyroid hormone therapy.

L-T_4 is considered a safe and effective replacement treatment for hypothyroid pregnant patients and is not teratogenic. A large population-based case-control study found that only 12 babies were born with major malformations to mothers with a history of hypothyroidism who were being treated with thyroid hormones during pregnancy.[8] These cases had no homogenous pattern of defects.

It is generally accepted that severe maternal hypothyroidism during the second trimester can result in irreversible neurologic deficits. Maternal hypothyroxinemia (fT_4 below the lowest 10th percentile and TSH within the reference range of 0.15 to 2.0 mU/L) at later stages can lead to less severe, and partially reversible, fetal brain damage. Even partial treatment of maternal hypothyroidism during pregnancy appears to be beneficial for offspring.[6] A recent cohort study found that infant neurodevelopment was not adversely affected by hypothyroxinemia during the first trimester if fT_4 concentrations were subsequently corrected.[9] Should we then treat all pregnant women with high TSH levels but no clinical hypothyroidism? We believe this decision must await results of randomized controlled trials of treatment.

DOSE ADJUSTMENT OF L-T$_4$ DURING PREGNANCY

Several studies have now confirmed that L-T$_4$ requirements in most women with existing hypothyroidism increase substantially during pregnancy. Absorption of T$_4$ occurs in the small intestine; it can absorb from 50% to 80% of the dose.[10] An empty stomach improves absorption. Sucralfate, cholestyramine resin, and aluminum hydroxide can interfere with L-T$_4$ absorption. Concomitant administration of drugs that induce hepatic cytochrome P450 (CYP) enzymes, mainly CYP3A4, such as phenytoin, carbamazepine, and rifampin, enhance biliary excretion of L-T$_4$. Hormonal and physiologic changes could indicate a need to adjust dosages during pregnancy.

Special attention should be paid to prenatal vitamins because they contain iron and calcium, both of which potently inhibit absorption of L-T$_4$.[11,12] A recent study found L-T$_4$ dosage adjustments were not required if prenatal vitamins were taken 4 hours after ingesting L-T$_4$.[13]

THERAPEUTIC DRUG MONITORING OF L-T$_4$

Because adverse effects for both mother and baby are not due to high serum TSH per se but to low free T$_4$ concentrations, decisions regarding treatment should be based on serum free T$_4$ concentrations rather than on serum TSH concentrations.[14] If the L-T$_4$ dose was increased during pregnancy, it should be reduced gradually after delivery and thyroid function evaluated repeatedly.

LEVOTHYROXINE AND BREASTFEEDING

The quantity of thyroid hormone transferred into human milk is too low to affect plasma thyroid hormone levels in neonates.[15] The American Academy of Pediatrics considers L-T$_4$ compatible with breast-feeding and has reported that no observable change is seen in nursing infants whose mothers are taking L-T$_4$.[16]

REFERENCES

1. Hollowell JG, Staehling NW, Flanders WD, et al. Serum TSH, T(4), and thyroid antibodies in the United States population (1988 to 1994): National Health and Nutrition Examination Survey (NHANES III). *J Clin Endocrinol Metab* 2002;87:489–499.

2. Allan WC, Haddow JE, Palomaki GE, Williams JR, et al. Maternal thyroid deficiency and pregnancy complications: implications for population screening. *J Med Screen* 2000;7:127–130.

3. Glinoer D. Management of hypo- and hyperthyroidism during pregnancy. *Growth Horm IGF Res* 2003;13(Suppl. A):S45–S54.

4. Contempre B, Jauniaux E, Culvo R, et al. Detection of thyroid hormones in human embryonic cavities during the first trimester of pregnancy. *J Clin Endocrinol Metab* 1993;77:1719–1722.

5. Lavado-Autric R, Auso E, Garcia-Velasco JV, et al. Early maternal hypothyroxinemia alters histogenesis and cerebral cortex cytoarchitecture of the progeny. *J Clin Invest* 2003;111:1073–1082.

6. Haddow JE, Palomaki GE, Allan WC, et al. Maternal thyroid deficiency during pregnancy and subsequent neuropsychological development of the child. *N Engl J Med* 1999;341:549–555.

7. Pop VJ, Kuijpens JL, van Baar AL, et al. Low maternal free thyroxine concentrations during early pregnancy are associated with impaired psychomotor development in infancy. *Clin Endocrinol* 1999;50:149–155.

8. Khoury MJ, Becerra JE, d'Almada PJ. Maternal thyroid disease and risk of birth defects in offspring: a population-based case-control study. *Paediatr Perinat Epidemiol* 1989;3:402–420.

9. Pop VJ, Brouwers EP, Vader HL, et al. Maternal hypothyroxinaemia during early pregnancy and subsequent child development: a 3-year follow-up study. *Clin Endocrinol* 2003;59:282–288.

10. Hays MT. Localization of human thyroxine absorption. *Thyroid* 1991;1:241–248.

11. Campbell NR, Hasinoff BB, Stalts H, et al. Ferrous sulfate reduces thyroxine efficacy in patients with hypothyroidism. *Ann Intern Med* 1992;117:1010–1013.

12. Singh N, Singh PN, Hershman JM. Effect of calcium carbonate on the absorption of levothyroxine. *JAMA* 2000;283:2822–2825.

13. Chopra IJ, Baber K. Treatment of primary hypothyroidism during pregnancy: is there an increase in thyroxine dose requirement in pregnancy? *Metabolism* 2003;52:122–128.

14. Poppe K, Glinoer D. Thyroid autoimmunity and hypothyroidism before and during pregnancy. *Human Reprod Update* 2003;9:149–161.

15. Van Wassenaer AG, Stulp MR, Valianpour F, et al. The quantity of thyroid hormone in human milk is too low to influence plasma thyroid hormone levels in the very preterm infant. *Clin Endocrinol* 2002;56:621–627.

16. American Academy of Pediatrics, Committee on Drugs. The transfer of drugs and other chemicals into human milk. *Pediatrics* 2001;108:776–789.

CHAPTER 34

EFFECTS OF PRENATAL EXPOSURE TO MARIJUANA

Eran Kozer, MD
Gideon Koren, MD, FRCPC

QUESTION

I am treating a 27-year-old woman who is now in her 10th week of pregnancy. She smokes marijuana two to three times a week, but does not use other drugs. She also smokes 20 cigarettes a day. I am concerned about the effects of marijuana exposure on her baby.

Answer

It is not always possible to isolate the effect of marijuana exposure from other possible confounders on pregnancy outcome. Although marijuana is not an established human teratogen, recent well-conducted studies suggest it might have subtle negative effects on neurobehavioural outcomes, including sleep disturbances, impaired visual problem solving, hyperactivity, impassivity, inattention, and increased delinquency.

Marijuana is a drug prepared from the plant *Cannabis sativa*. Its contains more than 400 chemicals including tetrahydrocannabinol (THC), its psychoactive component, which is rapidly absorbed from the lungs into the bloodstream and is metabolized primarily by the liver. Prolonged fetal exposure can occur if the mother is a regular user because THC crosses the placenta and because detectable levels can be found in various tissues up to 30 days after a single use.[1]

Trying to assess the outcome of in utero exposure to marijuana is complex. In many of the studies on marijuana exposure and pregnancy outcome, women who consume marijuana also smoked tobacco, drank alcohol, or used other drugs. The effect of marijuana exposure cannot always be isolated from other possible confounders. These limitations should be kept in mind when prenatal exposure to marijuana is considered.

EFFECTS ON A FETUS

Birth weight   Several studies demonstrated a small reduction in birth weight associated with use of marijuana during pregnancy,[2,3] while others failed to show such an effect.[4] A recent meta-analysis combined the results from 10 different studies on maternal cannabis use and birth weight[5] and showed only weak association between maternal cannabis use and birth weight. The largest reduction in mean birth weight for any cannabis use was 48 g (95% confidence interval [CI] 83 to 14 g). Cannabis use at least four times a day was associated with a larger reduction of 131 g (95% CI 52 to 209 g) in mean birth weight. The authors concluded that there is inadequate evidence that cannabis, at the amount typically consumed by pregnant women, causes low birth weight.

Teratogenicity   Marijuana has not been implicated as a human teratogen. No homogeneous pattern of malformation has been observed that could be considered characteristic of intrauterine marijuana exposure.[6] Among 202 infants exposed to marijuana prenatally, the rate of serious malformations was no higher than the rate among infants whose mothers did not use marijuana.[3]

Postnatal mortality   The mortality rate during the first 2 years of life was determined in 2964 infants. About 44% of the infants tested positive for drugs: 30.5% tested positive for cocaine, 20.2% for opiates, and 11.4% for cannabinoids. Mortality rates among the cannabinoid-positive group and the drug-negative group were not significantly different $(P > .3)$.[7]

Risk of childhood malignancy   A case-control study assessed in utero and postnatal exposures to drugs in 204 children with acute nonlymphoblastic leukemia.[8] An 11-fold risk $(P = .003)$ was found for maternal use of marijuana just before or during pregnancy. These findings should be interpreted cautiously because the rate of marijuana exposure in the control group was less than 1%. This rate is much lower than the 9% to 27% rate reported by others,[2–4] and might represent recall or reporting bias in this group. Such bias could increase the odds ratio (OR) associated with the exposure. In addition to the limitations of this study, another study could not confirm such an association.[9]

Another case-control study found an increased risk for rhab-domyosarcoma among children exposed to marijuana in utero.[10] In this study, it was impossible to differentiate between the effects of other agents on outcome because many women consumed marijuana with other drugs.

Current data are inconclusive, and further studies are needed to determine whether childhood malignancy is a true risk for fetuses exposed to marijuana.

Neurodevelopmental effects   Short- and long-term neurode-velopmental effects of prenatal exposure to marijuana are not clear. Because many women who use marijuana during pregnancy also use other illicit drugs, there are methodologic difficulties in interpreting the effects. In many studies, it is also difficult to isolate the effect of marijuana from other confounders, such as socioeconomic status, family structure, and mother's personality. Despite these limitations, evidence suggests that marijuana exposure during pregnancy has adverse fetal effects.

Sleep disturbances at 3 years of age were more common among offspring of women who used marijuana during pregnancy compared with controls.[11] The two groups were similar in maternal age, race, income, education, and maternal use of alcohol, nicotine, and other substances during the first trimester.

Child behavior was assessed at 10 years of age in 635 children from low-income families. Prenatal exposure to marijuana was associated with hyperactivity, impassivity, inattention, and increased delinquency.[12] In this cohort, women who used marijuana differed significantly from those who did not in many confounders that could affect child development. Although investigators tried to control for these variables, differences in behavior might be partially explained by other unrecognized confounders. In another study of one hundred forty six 9- to 12-year-old children, prenatal exposure to marijuana was not associated with intelligence, memory, or attention deficits.[13] The study showed prenatal exposure to marijuana is associated with poorer visual problem solving.

An example of the difficulties associated with assessing neurobehavioural outcomes after in utero exposure to marijuana comes from Jamaica. A study was conducted in an area where marijuana use is very common, and women who use large doses of marijuana are better educated and more independent than women who consume small doses of marijuana. At the age of 1 month, infants of heavy marijuana-using mothers had better scores on autonomic stability, quality of alertness, irritability, and self-regulation and were judged to be more rewarding for caregivers.[14] The authors suggested that these differences related to the characteristics of the mothers using marijuana.

It is possible, though, that neurobehavioural effects associated with in utero exposure to marijuana, which were observed in studies conducted in western countries, are partially related to the socioeconomic, behavioral, and psychological characteristics of women who consume marijuana during pregnancy and not to the exposure itself.

Marijuana is probably the most common illicit drug used during pregnancy.[15] Taking into account the large number of infants with prenatal exposure to marijuana, even a small influence on neurobehavioural parameters could have a noticeable effect on public health.

MARIJUANA AND BREASTFEEDING

Tetrahydrocannabinol is transferred into breast milk and levels can be up to eight times higher than in the mother's bloodstream.[16] Exposure to marijuana through breast milk might delay infants' motor development.[17] The American Academy of Pediatrics considers use of marijuana as a contraindication for breastfeeding.[18] It is advisable to abstain from all use of THC while breastfeeding.

REFERENCES

1. Jones RT. Human effects: an overview. *NIDA Res Monogr* 1980;31: 54–80.
2. Hatch EE, Bracken MB. Effect of marijuana use in pregnancy on fetal growth. *Am J Epidemiol* 1986;124(6):986–993.
3. Zuckerman B, Frank DA, Hingson R, et al. Effects of maternal marijuana and cocaine use on fetal growth. *N Engl J Med* 1989;320(12):762–768.
4. Shiono PH, Klebanoff MA, Nugent RP, et al. The impact of cocaine and marijuana use on low birth weight and preterm birth: a multicenter study. *Am J Obstet Gynecol* 1995;172(1 Pt. 1):19–27.
5. English DR, Hulse GK, et al. Maternal cannabis use and birth weight: a meta-analysis. *Addiction* 1997;92(11):1553–1560.
6. Briggs GG, Freeman RK, Yaffe SK, eds. Drugs in pregnancy and lactation. Baltimore, MD: Williams & Wilkins; 1998:647–657.
7. Ostrea EM Jr, Ostrea AR, Simpson PM. Mortality within the first 2 years in infants exposed to cocaine, opiate, or cannabinoid during gestation. *Pediatrics* 1997;100(1):79–83.

8. Robison LL, Buckley JD, Daigle AE, et al. Maternal drug use and risk of childhood nonlymphoblastic leukemia among offspring. An epidemiologic investigation implicating marijuana (a report from the Childrens Cancer Study Group). *Cancer* 1989;63(10):1904–1911.

9. van Duijn CM, Steensel-Moll HA, Coebergh JW, et al. Risk factors for childhood acute non-lymphocytic leukemia: an association with maternal alcohol consumption during pregnancy? *Cancer Epidemiol Biomarkers Prev* 1994;3(6):457–460.

10. Grufferman S, Schwartz AG, Ruymann FB, et al. Parents' use of cocaine and marijuana and increased risk of rhabdomyosarcoma in their children. *Cancer Causes Control* 1993;4(3):217–224.

11. Dahl RE, Scher MS, Williamson DE, et al. A longitudinal study of prenatal marijuana use. Effects on sleep and arousal at age 3 years. *Arch Pediatr Adolesc Med* 1995;149(2):145–150.

12. Goldschmidt L, Day NL, Richardson GA. Effects of prenatal marijuana exposure on child behavior problems at age 10. *Neurotoxicol Teratol* 2000;22(3):325–336.

13. Fried PA, Watkinson B. Visuoperceptual functioning differs in 9- to 12-year olds prenatally exposed to cigarettes and marihuana. *Neurotoxicol Teratol* 2000;22(1):11–20.

14. Dreher MC, Nugent K, Hudgins R. Prenatal marijuana exposure and neonatal outcomes in Jamaica: an ethnographic study. *Pediatrics* 1994; 93(2):254–260.

15. Feng T. Substance abuse in pregnancy. *Curr Opin Obstet Gynecol* 1993;5(1):16–23.

16. Perez-Reyes M, Wall ME. Presence of delta9-tetrahydrocannabinol in human milk. *N Engl J Med* 1982;307(13):819–820.

17. Ito S. Drug therapy for breast-feeding women. *N Engl J Med* 2000; 343(2):118–126.

18. American Academy of Pediatrics Committee on Drugs. The transfer of drugs and other chemicals into human milk. *Pediatrics* 1994;93(1): 137–150.

MARIJUANA USE AND BREASTFEEDING

Myla Moretti, MSc
Gideon Koren, MD, FRCPC

QUESTION

One of my breastfeeding patients is using marijuana to combat chronic pain. Is it safe for her to breastfeed?

Answer

Lactating mothers should refrain from consuming cannabinoids. Advising mothers to discontinue breastfeeding if they cannot stop using cannabinoids must incorporate the known risks of formula feeding. Cannabinoid exposure through milk has not been shown to increase neonatal risk, but there are no appropriate studies of this. In every case, nursing babies should be closely monitored.

Despite abundant recreational use of cannabinoids by women of reproductive age, very little is known about marijuana use and lactation. The Motherisk Program's Alcohol and Substance Use Helpline receives about three calls a week regarding use of marijuana by nursing mothers for recreational purposes or for health issues, such as depression, anxiety, or pain. Questions come from nursing mothers themselves, friends, relatives, and health care providers concerned about exposure of breastfed babies.

Marijuana is a crude preparation of the leaves and flowering tops of *Cannabis sativa*. It is most commonly smoked and inhaled, but it can also be ingested orally. The psychological effects of marijuana include euphoria, relaxation, slowed thinking and reaction time, altered perception, impaired coordination and motor performance, poor short-term memory, impaired attention and judgment, panic attacks, anxiety, dizziness, and general difficulty expressing even simple thoughts in words. Other effects include increased heart rate, reddened eyes, dizziness, dry mouth, increased appetite, nausea, respiratory disorder, and immune system dysfunction.[1–6]

Delta-9-tetrahydrocannabinol (THC) is the principal psychoactive compound in marijuana. In addition to THC, marijuana smoke contains more than 150 other compounds.[6] The THC is absorbed from the gastrointestinal tract and lungs and, being highly lipophilic, is rapidly distributed to the brain and fat tissue and extensively bound to plasma proteins (97%). The THC is metabolized in the liver and has an elimination half-life of 20 to 36 hours.[7] In chronic users, its half-life could be as long as 4 days because it is stored in body fat; it can be detected for up to a month after last use. It is excreted in urine and feces over a prolonged period.

The passage of THC into breast milk has not been extensively studied. A study by Perez-Reyes and Wall in 1982 suggested that THC is excreted into human breast milk in moderate amounts.[8] Based on their findings, 0.8% of the weight-adjusted maternal intake of one joint would be ingested by an infant in one feeding[7] (i.e., the baby would receive 0.8% of its mother's dose/kg). In heavy users, the milk-to-plasma ratio (i.e., levels in milk vs. levels in maternal blood) was as high as 8:1.[8] Animal studies suggest that marijuana can decrease the amount of milk produced by suppressing prolactin production and possibly through a direct effect on the mammary glands. There are no human data to corroborate these observations.

In 1990, a study by Astley and Little suggested that exposure to THC through breast milk in the first month of life could result in decreased motor development at the age of one year.[9] No studies have adequately addressed the effects on long-term neurodevelopment. Lethargy, less frequent feeding, and shorter feeding times are other observations reported after babies' exposure to THC through breast milk.[10] A mother's ability to nurse and care for her child might be compromised because marijuana can affect mood and judgment.

Breast milk is the best food for babies. It contains appropriate amounts of carbohydrates, proteins, fats, minerals, vitamins, and hormones as well as maternal antibodies. Psychologically, breastfeeding facilitates bonding between mother and child.

With chronic use, THC can accumulate in human breast milk to high concentrations.[8] Because a baby's brain is still forming, THC could theoretically affect brain development. It is also important to avoid environmental exposure to maternal marijuana smoke. Nursing mothers should be referred to appropriate services for counseling.

REFERENCES

1. American Academy of Pediatrics. Marijuana: a continuing concern for pediatricians. *Pediatrics* 1999;104:982–985.
2. Thomas H. Psychiatric symptoms in cannabis users. *Br J Psychiatry* 1993;163:141–149.
3. Naditch MP, Alker PC, Joffe P. Individual differences and setting as determinants of acute adverse reactions to psychoactive drugs. *J Nerv Ment Dis* 1975;161:326–335.
4. Chait LD, Pierri J. Effects of smoked marijuana on human performance: a critical review. In: Murphy I, Bartke A, eds. *Marijuana/Cannabinoids: Neurobiology and Neurophysiology*. Boca Raton, FL: CRC Press; 1992: 387–423.
5. Hubbard JR, Franco SE, Onavaivi ES. Marijuana: medical implications. *Am Fam Physician* 1999;60:2583–2593.
6. Gold MS. The pharmacology of marijuana. In: Graham AW, Schultz TK, eds. *Principles of Addiction Medicine*. Chevy Chase, MD: American Society of Addiction Medicine 1998:163–171.
7. Bennett PN. Cannabis. In: Bennett PN and the WHO Working Group, eds.. *Drugs and Human Lactation*. 2nd ed. Amsterdam, Holl: Elsevier; 1997.
8. Perez-Reyes M, Wall ME. Presence of delta-9-tetrahydrocannabinol in human milk. *N Engl J Med* 1982;307:819–820.
9. Astley S, Little RE. Maternal marijuana use during lactation and infant development at one year. *Neurotoxicol Teratol* 1990;12:161–168.
10. Committee on Nutritional Status During Pregnancy and Lactation, Institute of Medicine. *Illegal Drugs*. Washington, DC: National Academy Press; 1991.

METFORMIN USE DURING THE FIRST TRIMESTER OF PREGNANCY: IS IT SAFE?

Gideon Koren, MD, FRCPC
Cameron J. Gilbert, MSc

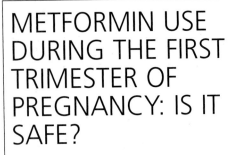

QUESTION

A pregnant patient with polycystic ovary syndrome (PCOS) asked me whether continuing metformin, which she was taking to treat infertility before her pregnancy, was safe for her fetus. She had heard that metformin is a "drug for diabetes." How safe is it to take metformin during the first trimester of pregnancy and beyond?

Answer

Despite the traditional response that all oral hypoglycemic agents are absolutely contraindicated during pregnancy,[1-3] evidence that metformin is probably safe during the first trimester of pregnancy and beyond is accumulating. Results of a recent meta-analysis by the Motherisk Program showed no increase in incidence of major malformations and a potential protective effect in this patient population.

PCOS is defined by the presence of oligo-ovulation or anovulation in combination with hyperandrogenism. Between 5% and 7% of women of reproductive age have PCOS,[4] making it the most common cause of anovulatory infertility.[5]

Metformin is currently approved by the U.S. Food and Drug Administration for treatment of type 2 diabetes.[6] The most current product monograph still lists pregnancy as a contraindication to the use of metformin; however, in both Canada and the United States, its off-label use in treatment of infertility caused by PCOS is growing.

Metformin is known to facilitate conception in women who have oligomenorrhoea and PCOS.[7,8] Recent studies have suggested that metformin use during pregnancy decreases the high incidence of spontaneous abortion associated with PCOS (30% to 50%)[9] and with gestational diabetes (31% in untreated women vs. 3% in treated women).[10]

ANIMAL STUDIES

Whether metformin causes teratogenicity in animals is controversial. Some animal studies found no evidence of teratogenicity at doses as high as 600 mg/kg daily.[11] One study showed that metformin at doses similar to clinical in vivo levels had no direct toxic effects on mouse embryo development.[12] Another study showed that, although exposure to both biguanides, phenformin and metformin, were associated with embryo death, phenformin has greater toxicity in mouse whole embryo culture, suggesting that metformin might be safer to use during pregnancy.[13] Other studies, however, have suggested that metformin induces a low incidence of malformations in rats.[14] For women taking metformin for PCOS, the question of teratogenicity remains challenging because it is difficult to clarify whether the teratogenic potential is subsequent to poor glycemic control or subsequent to the direct actions of the oral hypoglycemic drug itself.

FIRST-TRIMESTER EXPOSURE

The Motherisk Program recently conducted a retrospective cohort study on pregnancy outcome among women with PCOS[15] and a meta-analysis of all published studies with data on pregnancy outcomes with respect to major malformations.[16] In the retrospective cohort study, 72 PCOS patients exposed to metformin were compared with 48 PCOS patients who conceived without metformin in five different fertility clinics. The prevalence of major malformations was similar in the two groups. The metformin group had a higher prevalence of multiple pregnancies and prematurity. Prematurity is a substantial confounder of concomitant use of other fertility drugs.[15]

Results of the meta-analysis are encouraging. In the five studies included in the statistical analysis, there was no increase in the rate of major malformations, and in fact, metformin might actually have a protective effect in women with PCOS. In the treated group, there were three malformations among 172 babies (1.7%); in the control group, there were 17 malformations among 235 babies (7.2%). The odds ratio was 0.50 in favor of treatment.[16]

In summary, no evidence currently in the literature shows that use of metformin in women with PCOS is associated with increased risk of malformations. Most of the studies applicable to PCOS restricted exposure to the first trimester, i.e., metformin was discontinued as soon as pregnancy was diagnosed. Evidence beyond the first trimester is anecdotal at this point. Large well-controlled studies of humans are needed. For women with non-insulin-dependent diabetes mellitus, insulin is still considered the treatment of choice during pregnancy, although glyburide has been shown not to cross the human placenta.[17,18]

REFERENCES

1. Hellmuth E, Damm P, Molsted-Pedersen L. Oral hypoglycaemic agents in 118 diabetic pregnancies. *Diabet Med* 2000;17(7):507–511.
2. Piacquadio K, Hollingsworth DR, Murphy H. Effects of in-utero exposure to oral hypoglycaemic drugs. *Lancet* 1991;338(8771):866–869.
3. Meltzer S, Leiter L, Daneman D, et al. 1998 clinical practice guidelines for the management of diabetes in Canada. Canadian Diabetes Association. *CMAJ* 1998;159(Suppl. 8):S1–S29.
4. Barbieri RL. Metformin for the treatment of polycystic ovary syndrome. *Obstet Gynecol* 2003;101(4):785–793.
5. Danaif A. Insulin resistance and the polycystic ovary syndrome: mechanism and implications for pathogenesis. *Endocr Rev* 1997;8:774–800.
6. U.S. Food and Drug Administration. Metformin product monograph. Washington, DC: United States Food and Drug Administration; 2000. Available at: http://www.fda.gov/cder/foi/label/2000/21202lbl.pdf. Accessed 2005 December 20.
7. Ben Haroush A, Yogev Y, Fisch B. Insulin resistance and metformin in polycystic ovary syndrome. *Eur J Obstet Gynecol Reprod Biol* 2004; 115(2):125–133.
8. McCarthy EA, Walker SP, McLachlan K, et al. Metformin in obstetric and gynecologic practice: a review. *Obstet Gynecol Surv* 2004;59(2): 118–127.
9. Glueck CJ, Phillips H, Cameron D, et al. Continuing metformin throughout pregnancy in women with polycystic ovary syndrome appears to safely reduce first-trimester spontaneous abortion: a pilot study. *Fertil Steril* 2001;75(1):46–52.
10. Glueck CJ, Wang P, Kobayashi S, et al. Metformin therapy throughout pregnancy reduces the development of gestational diabetes in women with polycystic ovary syndrome. *Fertil Steril* 2002;77(3):520–525.

11. Briggs GG, Freeman RK, Yaffe SJ. *Drugs in Pregnancy and Lactation*. Philadelphia, PA: Lippincott, Williams & Wilkins; 2002.

12. Bedaiwy MA, Miller KF, Goldberg JM, et al. Effect of metformin on mouse embryo development. *Fertil Steril* 2001;76(5):1078–1079.

13. Denno KM, Sadler TW. Effects of the biguanide class of oral hypoglycemic agents on mouse embryogenesis. *Teratology* 1994;49(4):260–266.

14. Schardein JL. *Chemically Induced Birth Defects*. New York, NY: Marcel Dekker Inc.; 2000.

15. Gargaun S, Ryan E, Greenblatt E, et al. Pregnancy outcome in women with polycystic ovary syndrome exposed to metformin [abstract]. *Can J Clin Pharmacol* 2003;10(3):e149. Available at: http://www.pulsus.com/clin-pha/10_03/cscp_ed.htm. Accessed 2006 January 6.

16. Gilbert C, Koren G. Pregnancy outcome following first-trimester exposure to metformin: a meta-analysis [abstract]. *Can J Clin Pharmacol* 2005;12(1):e125. Available from: http://www.cjcp.ca/pdf/Second_ Congress_Abstracts_e41-e149.pdf. Accessed 2006 January 6.

17. Koren G. Glyburide and fetal safety; transplacental pharmacokinetic considerations. *Reprod Toxicol* 2001;15(3):227–229.

18. Langer O, Conway DL, Berkus MD, et al. A comparison of glyburide and insulin in women with gestational diabetes mellitus. *N Engl J Med* 2000; 343(16):1134–1138.

CHAPTER 37

IS THE FETUS SAFE WHEN SPERMICIDES FAIL?

Gideon Koren, MD, FRCPC

QUESTION

One of my patients had been using spermicides for contraception. She discovered she was 8 weeks pregnant despite using "foam." Because spermicides kill sperm, how can we be sure that they do not damage the sperm that participate in fertilization?

Answer

The literature contains several reports associating spermicides with adverse fetal outcomes. This has led to much comment and litigation, particularly in the United States. Huggins et al.[1] suggest three possible mechanisms of action if spermicides are teratogenic: the spermicide could be absorbed through the vaginal wall before conception and damage the ovum; sperm could be damaged, but not deactivated, by the spermicide and subsequently could fertilize the ovum; and the spermicide could be absorbed after fertilization and directly damage the embryo. A fourth possibility suggested by Bracken and Vita[2] was that sperm might transport spermicide to the ovum where it could interfere with the mother's genetic material.

Studies have produced conflicting results. One statistical method for obtaining an overall quantitative estimate of the effect of a drug on reproduction, especially when conflict exists, is meta-analysis.[3] This technique has been widely used in such cases and is gaining increased popularity in medicine. We recently studied the relationship between mother's use of spermicides and subsequent adverse fetal outcomes using meta-analysis.[4] Nine studies investigating teratogenicity met the inclusion criteria; the Mantel-Haenszel summary odds ratio was 1.02 (95% confidence interval [CI] 0.78 to 1.32). The χ^2 analyses were 0.10

for significance from unity ($P = 0.748$) and 8.73 for homogeneity of effects ($P = 0.365$). Studies comparing specific abnormalities with other abnormalities also indicated no association (odds ratio = 0.96; 95% CI 0.72 to 1.28). Studies investigating other adverse events (spontaneous abortion, stillbirth, low fetal weight, prematurity, increased incidence of female births) also had negative results. Cohen's D, the overall effect size as determined by Tukey's method, was –0.001 (95% CI –0.018 to 0.017). These results indicate that mothers' use of spermicides is not associated with adverse fetal outcomes.

Because rates of spontaneous adverse reproductive outcomes are very low, most studies that attempt to establish relationships between potential teratogens and outcome cannot recruit enough cases to reach an adequate level of statistical power. Physicians and scientists, trying to determine whether a drug or chemical is a potential human teratogen, must often decide which of the studies that present opposing results is more credible.

Meta-analysis allows date from different studies to be combined, so that appropriate statistical power can be achieved. The main criticism of the method is that "good" studies are combined with "bad" studies with each receiving equal weight. However, when meta-analysis is performed appropriately, the problem dissipates. If a blinded reviewer includes or excludes studies according to preset criteria, such methodologic issues are minimized.

In the litigious atmosphere around health care today, we must develop and crystallize scientific tools powerful enough to disqualify the devastating effects of invalid cases presented to juries. Classically, studies presented by plaintiffs (generally parents of malformed children) must stand against conflicting studies presented by defendants (generally pharmaceutical manufacturers, physicians, or both). Lawyers, judges, and physicians cannot be expected to be able to evaluate single studies in isolation from the statistical context of all available evidence. Meta-analysis is the only approach that combines such data and derives an overall estimate of risk.

Beyond its inherent advantages, meta-analysis also forces reviewers to evaluate the methods and results of each study closely to determine acceptability for inclusion. The value of using blinded reviewers is self-evident.

The meta-analysis in this study showed that mothers' use of spermicides is not associated with fetal malformations or any other reported abnormal fetal outcomes. We hope that these results, on the basis of all available studies, will help stop the flood of unnecessary and unfounded litigation. We also hope that meta-analysis will become the standard for evaluating reproductive outcome after exposure to drugs, chemicals, radiation, and infections during pregnancy.

REFERENCES

1. Huggins G, Vessy M, Flavel R, et al. Vaginal spermicides and outcome of pregnancy: finding in a large cohort study. *Contraception* 1982;25: 219–230.
2. Bracken MB, Vita K. Frequency of non-hormonal contraception around conception and association with congenital malformations in offspring. *Am J Epidemiol* 1983;117:281–291.
3. Einarson TR, Leeder JS, Koren G. A method for meta-analysis of epidemiologic studies. *Drug Intell Clin Pharm* 1988;22:813–824.
4. Einarson TR, Koren G, Mattice D. Maternal spermicide use and adverse reproductive outcome: A meta-analysis. *Am J Obstet Gynecol* 1990;162: 655–660.

CHAPTER 38

ACID-SUPPRESSING DRUGS DURING PREGNANCY

Gideon Koren, MD, FRCPC

QUESTION

One of my patients suffers from a severe form of gastroesophageal reflux and regurgitation. She has just conceived. She has tried to manage her conditions with an antacid agent, but has not been successful. I hesitate to put her on an acid-suppressing drug. What is your recommendation?

Answer

Acid-suppressing drugs, mainly H2-blockers and omeprazole, do not appear to cause measurable teratogenic risk in humans. Given the much wider experience with ranitidine than with omeprazole, however, they should remain the drugs of choice at present. Rapid accumulation of data on omeprazole and initial reassuring results could mean we will add this drug to first-line therapy in the future.

Gastroesophageal reflux is a common and troublesome disorder during pregnancy. Heartburn affects 30% to 50% of all pregnant women and tends to worsen as pregnancy advances. Lower esophageal sphincter pressure decreases and the sphincter's adaptive responses can be inhibited. It is unclear whether estrogen, progesterone, or both influence sphincter tonus.[1] Upper abdominal pain, regurgitation, and heartburn can be severe, and therapy might be mandatory. Some women restrict their meals to once daily due to severe postprandial symptoms; others are forced to sleep upright all night.

The main goal of treatment is to relieve symptoms. Effective acid-suppressing drugs are available now for treating peptic and gastric ulcer, reflux esophagitis, and Zollinger-Ellison syndrome. Data on the safety of acid-suppressing drugs during human pregnancy are, however, scarce. To address this issue, we searched MEDLINE and EMBASE for literature published up to 1997 with omeprazole and

H2-antagonists as key words (MeSH exploded) matched with *pregnancy* and *abnormality, drug-induced* (MeSH exploded).

SAFETY OF H$_2$-BLOCKER USE IN EARLY PREGNANCY

All H$_2$-blockers cross the human placenta. Animal reproductive toxicology studies, however, failed to show that any of the H$_2$-blockers were teratogenic.[2] Of particular note, no consistent animal data prove that cimetidine has antiandrogenic effects in utero. Neither postmarketing surveillance conducted by North American drug manufacturers, nor five anecdotal reports of cimetidine or five of ranitidine exposure during the first trimester, nor record linkage studies[3] and the Michigan Medicaid Surveillance Study (conducted from 1985 to 1992 examining cimetidine in 480 patients, ranitidine in 516 patients, and famotidine in 33 patients) have reported evidence of teratogenicity.

In the only prospective study on the topic,[4] 178 (77.4%) of a possible 230 women who called the Motherisk Program about gestational H$_2$-blocker use were recruited. Their pregnancy outcomes were compared with those of 178 controls matched for age, smoking, and heavy alcohol consumption. Most patients ingested ranitidine (71%, mean dose 258±99 mg/day); others took cimetidine (16%, 487±389 mg/day), famotidine (8%, 32±10 mg/year), and nizatidine (5%, 283±139 mg/day). The primary indication was heartburn (41%), followed by peptic ulcer disease (30%), epigastric pain (17%), and other conditions (12%), which included prophylaxis against mucosal ulceration. No increase in major malformations was found following first-trimester exposure to H$_2$-blockers: 3 of 142 (2.1%) H$_2$-blocker users had infants with major malformations compared with 5 of 143 (3.5%) controls ($P = 0.55$; mean difference 1.4% [95% confidence interval 5.2±2.4]).

Therefore, no evidence indicates that H$_2$-blocker exposure during the first trimester is associated with increased risk of major malformations above the baseline risk of 1% to 3% in all pregnancies. For patients receiving long-term therapy, however, it might be prudent to review the indication for the medication, especially in the light of recent evidence showing a strong etiologic role for *Helicobacter pylori* infection in gastric and duodenal ulceration; the role of this infection in non-ulcer dyspepsia is uncertain.[5] Various regimens have been recommended for treating *H. pylori*.[6]

SAFETY OF H$_2$-BLOCKER USE LATER IN PREGNANCY

Clinical diagnosis of gastroesophageal reflux is straightforward when a patient describes retrosternal burning that radiates up to the neck, often after lying down. Given that complications of reflux are uncommon in pregnancy, the therapeutic goal is symptom relief.

Lifestyle modifications should be recommended first for all patients with uncomplicated reflux. Although these measures have not been proven effective by clinical trials, they are safe, inexpensive, and appear to be effective for many patients. Such measures include elevating the head of the bed, avoiding bedtime snacks or late meals, choosing low-fat foods, quitting smoking, and controlling symptoms with antacids or alginic acid.

There is little information on the effect on fetal or neonatal outcomes of taking H$_2$-blockers later in pregnancy. In the Motherisk study, no aspects of pregnancy outcome (including prematurity and low birth weight) or neonatal health differed between H$_2$-blocker users and controls, even when outcomes of only the 22% of neonates exposed to H$_2$-blockers at delivery were analyzed. Nor did the incidence of jaundice differ between groups (9.7% [16/164] of users vs. 14.9% [24/161] of controls, $P = 0.16$). Although hepatic and renal clearance of H$_2$-blockers can be slower in neonates, only one case of unexplained cholestatic jaundice has been reported following cimetidine exposure during the third trimester.[7] This must be interpreted in light of the obstetric anesthesia literature, which has documented no H$_2$-blocker-induced neonatal side effects when these drugs have been administered at term.[2] More studies are needed, however, to confirm the safety of these agents during late pregnancy.

Antisecretory agents, by comparison with most other classes of drugs, are remarkably well tolerated.[8] Reports of maternal anaphylactoid reactions to ranitidine[9,10] must be interpreted in this context.

SAFETY OF OMEPRAZOLE

Omeprazole, a proton pump inhibitor, has been shown to be very efficient for treating duodenal and gastric ulcer and is the drug of choice for reflux esophagitis.[11] Although it crosses the placenta, animal studies failed to show drug-induced teratogenicity following doses 250 to 500 times the recommended dose for humans.[12,13] Human data are scarce and consist of a few published case reports and spontaneous reports to the manufacturers.[14,15] In these reports, there was no consistency in type of abnormality reported or stage of pregnancy when the mother was exposed to omeprazole. The Motherisk Program conducted the first prospective cohort study. 113 pregnant women exposed to omeprazole showing no significant difference in the incidence of major malformations in their infants. The exposed and control women were similar in many ways, including gestational age at delivery, number of preterm deliveries, birth weight, method of delivery, and neonatal health problems.

Based on current information, we conclude that antisecretory drugs are safe during pregnancy. Because these drugs are both efficacious and devoid of serious side effects and because pregnant women suffer from gastroesophageal reflux quite often, we believe this information is reassuring.

REFERENCES

1. Baron TH, Ramirez B, Richter JE. Gastrointestinal motility disorders during pregnancy. *Ann Intern Med* 1993;118:366–375.
2. Briggs GG, Freeman RK, Yaffe SJ, eds. *Drugs in Pregnancy and Lactation.* 6th ed. Baltimore, MD: Williams & Wilkins; 2004.
3. Colin Jones DG, Langman MJS, Lawson DH, et al. Post-marketing surveillance of the safety of cimetidine: twelve-month morbidity report. *Q J Med* 1985;54(215):253–268.
4. Magee LA, Inocencion G, Kamboj L, et al. Safety of first trimester exposure to histamine H_2 blockers. *Dig Dis Sci* 1996;41(6):1145–1149.
5. Talley NJ. Modern management of dyspepsia. *Aust Fam Physician* 1996;25(1):47–52.
6. Drugs for treatment of peptic ulcers. *Med Lett Drugs Ther* 1997; 39(991):1–4.
7. Glade G, Saccar CL, Pereira GR. Cimetidine in pregnancy: apparent transient liver impairment in the newborn. *Am J Dis Child* 1980;134:87–88.
8. Smallwood RA, Berlin RG, Castagnoli N, et al. Safety of acid-suppressing drugs. *Dig Dis Sci* 1995;40(Suppl. 2):63S–80S.
9. Powell JA, Maycock EJ. Anaphylactoid reaction to ranitidine in an obstetric patient. *Anaesth Intensive Care* 1993;21(5):702–703.
10. Barry JE, Madan R, Hewitt PB. Anaphylactoid reaction to ranitidine in an obstetric patient. *Anaesthesia* 1992; 47(4):360–361.
11. Clissold SP, Campoli-Richard DM. Omeprazole—a preliminary review of its pharmacodynamics and pharmacokinetics properties, and therapeutic potential in peptic ulcer disease and Zollinger-Ellison syndrome. *Drugs* 1986;32:15–47.

12. Ekman L, Hansson E, Habu N, et al. Toxicological studies on omeprazole. *Scand J Gastroenterol Suppl* 1985; 20(Suppl. 108):53–69.

13. *Losec.* Product Monograph. Mississauga, Ont: Astra Pharm Inc; 1996.

14. Hollenz M. Omeprazole during pregnancy. A case report. *TW Gynekologie* 1992;5:235–236.

15. Harper MA, McVeigh JE, Thompson W, et al. Successful pregnancy in association with Zollinger-Ellison syndrome. *Am J Obstet Gynecol* 1995; 173:863–864.

16. Lalkin A, Loebstein R, Addis A, et al. The safety of omeprazole during pregnancy: a multicenter prospective controlled stydy. *Am J Obstet Glynecol* 1998;179:727–730.

CHAPTER 39

COUNSELING PREGNANT WOMEN WHO ARE TREATED WITH PAROXETINE

Adrienne Einarson RN
Gideon Koren MD, FRCPC

QUESTION

I have always reassured my patients that taking a Selective serotonin reuptake inhibitors (SSRI) in pregnancy would not increase their risk for having a child with a major malformation. However, I recently read the warning from Health Canada regarding the release of a study from Glaxo Smith Cline (GSK), stating that infants exposed to paroxetine may be at a higher risk of congenital malformations, specifically cardiovascular defects. Some of my peers heard about these pregnant patients who are taking paroxetine and called me to ask if they should stop taking it. What should I tell them?

Answer

The new warning is based on nonpeer review, unpublished studies. It ignored two published studies that failed to show such association, and no such association has been shown for SSRIs as a class. The data suggested that even if there is a risk, it is small. The warning does not disclose the details of the cardiovascular malformations in these studies. Many cases of ventricular septal defect, the most common cardiac malformation, resolve spontaneously. Concerned mothers to be, should know that beyond the first trimester a drug cannot cause cardiac malformation. Failure to treat depression during pregnancy can have significant negative ramifications for both mother and child, and it is the strongest predictor of postpartum depression.

To date, none of the SSRIs have been associated with an increased risk for major malformations, including cardiovascular anomalies.[1]

Recently, GSK released an advisory[2] which subsequently was incorporated in a Health Canada Advisory,[3] indicating that infants exposed to paroxetine at the time of organogenesis were at a higher risk of congenital malformations, particularly cardiovascular (ventricular septal) defects. This information was based on an unpublished, retrospective, epidemiologic study, conducted by GSK, as well as three abstracts presented at scientific conferences.

The GSK study claimed a prevalence of major malformations as a whole was 4% and for cardiovascular malformations it was 2%.[2] Alwan et al. presented a case control study that showed an increased risk of major malformations in general, but no association with cardiovascular defects.[4] Wogleus et al. claimed a small increase in cardiovascular malformations based on a prescription database study where it was not known whether pregnant women actually took the medication.[5] Finally, Diav-Citrin et al. presented a prospective comparative study, that also showed a small increase in the rates of cardiovascular defects (1.9%).[6] At the present time, these data are based on unpublished, non peer-reviewed studies. Therefore, one needs to be extremely careful in accepting them as scientific facts. It should be noted that cardiovascular malformations are common in the general population, occurring in approximately 1% of all births. In addition, we do not know the details of the cardiovascular malformations and some could be, in any of these preliminary reports, minor. For example, a large proportion of ventricular septal defects (of the muscular type) resolve spontaneously. The data suggest that even if there is a malformation risk it is of marginal magnitude. Of importance, this association has not been found with other SSRI drugs. To date there has been no evidence that in a class of drugs, only one agent is associated with an increased risk for birth defects while the others are not. This suggested association has not been found in previous published studies on paroxetine. Ericson et al. published a study which included 122 cases of embryonal exposure to paroxetine and there was no difference in the rates of cardiovascular defects between paroxetine and controls.[7] Similarly, Motherisk published a study of 267 women exposed to SSRIs where two cardiovascular defects were described. One of these occurred among 97 fetuses exposed to paroxetine, a similar rate to the other SSRIs (1/169).[8] Further, we have reanalyzed our recent meta-analysis of congenital anomalies with SSRIs as compared to controls[1] and could not detect an increased risk of cardiac malformation for SSRIs as a class. Last, a large case control study from Sweden has failed to show an association

TABLE 39-1
MOTHERISK GUIDELINES FOR MANAGING PREGNANT WOMEN ON
PAROXETINE AND OTHER SSRIs

- Ensure that diagnosis and symptoms warrant an antidepressant.
- Ensure that the woman is on an appropriate dose that controls her symptom. In late pregnancy many women need more of the medication.
- An ultrasound or fetal echocardiogram may detect cardiovascular malformations.
- Never discontinue the drug "cold turkey", rather taper it off.

between cardiac malformations and SSRI (Odds Ratio[OR] 0.95, 95% confidence interval[CI] 0.62-1.44).[9] Taken together, there are three peer-reviewed published studies showing no increased rates of cardiovascular malformations with paroxetine. One of the four recent unpublished reports also could not find increased risk of cardiovascular malformations whereas three had an apparent small risk.

Failure to treat depression during pregnancy can have significant negative ramifications for both mother and child, most notably, it is the strongest predictor of postpartum depression, which can sometimes have tragic consequences.[10]

As expected from such unbalanced reports, many women regrettably discontinued their Paxil even after the first trimester, when cardiac malformation cannot be produced. Women and their physicians should discuss this information and make an informed decision, whether or not to continue on this medication during pregnancy. As shown in Table 39-1, concerned patients can be offered ultrasound and echocardiogram which can rule out fetal cardiac problems in early pregnancy. Antidepressants should never be stopped abruptly as this can have serious ramifications for the mother.[11] If a woman does decide, following a discussion with her physician, that she wants to discontinue paroxetine, the drug should be slowly tapered off over a number of weeks.

REFERENCES

1. Einarson TR, Einarson A. Newer antidepressants in pregnancy and rates of major malformations: a meta-analysis of prospective comparative studies. *Pharmacoepidemiol Drug Saf.* 2005 Mar 1;[Epub ahead of print].
2. GSK Advisory October 2005. http://ctr.gsk.co.uk/welcome.asp.
3. Health Canada Advisory October 2005. http://hc-sc.gc.ca/dhp-mps/medeff/advisories-avis/prof/index e.html

4. Alwan S, Reefhuis J, Rasmussen S, et al. (Abstract) Maternal use of selective serotonin re-uptake inhibitors and risk for birth defects. *Birth Defects Research* (Part A): *Clinical and Molecular Teratology* 2005;731:291.

5. Wogleus P, Norgaard M, Muff Munk E, et al. (Abstract) Maternal use of selective serotonin reuptake inhibitors and risk of adverse pregnancy outcomes. *Pharmacoepidemiology and Drug Safety* 2005;14:143S.

6. Diav-Citrin, Ornoy A. Pregnancy outcome after gestation exposure to paroxetine: (Abstract). A prospective controlled cohort study. Teratology meeting. St. Petersburg, FL, June 2005.

7. Ericson A, Kallen B, Wilholm BE. Delivery outcome after the use of antidepressants in early pregnancy. *European Journal of Clinical Pharmacology* 1999;55:503–508.

8. Kulin NA, Pastuszak A, Sage S, et al. Pregnancy outcome following maternal use of the new selective serotonin reuptake inhibitors A prospective controlled multicenter study. *JAMA* 1998;279:609–610.

9. Kallen BA, Otterblad Olausson P. Maternal drug use in early pregnancy and infant cardiovascular defect. *Reprod Toxicol* 2003;17:255–261.

10. Beck CT. Postpartum depression predictors inventory revised. *Adv Neonatal care.* 2003 Feb;3(1):47–48.

11. Einarson A, Selby P, Koren G. Abrupt discontinuation of psychotropic drugs during pregnancy: fear of teratogenic risk and impact of counseling. *J Psychiatry Neurosci* 2001;(1):44–48.

DISCONTINUING ANTIDEPRESSANTS AND BENZODIAZEPINES UPON BECOMING PREGNANT

Adrienne Einarson, RN
Gideon Koren, MD, FRCPC

QUESTION

Two of my patients are planning to become pregnant. One is taking paroxetine and the other lorazepam. We have discussed what to do when they become pregnant and have decided they should stop taking these drugs as soon as pregnancy is confirmed. Is this the right decision?

Answer

The decision to discontinue these drugs during pregnancy should be based on scientific evidence rather than "hearsay" that women should not take psychotropic medications during pregnancy. Recent epidemiologic studies have documented the relative safety of these drugs, so women should not feel compelled to stop taking them when they become pregnant. If, after receiving appropriate evidence-based information, a woman decides to stop taking the drugs, they should be gradually tapered off to avoid abrupt discontinuation syndrome.

Depression and anxiety disorders are common among women of childbearing age, and these women are often prescribed antidepressants and benzodiazepines. Although many of these drugs have been found not to be teratogenic,[1-4] fear of taking them during pregnancy persists. For some reason, more fear appears to surround use of psychotropic drugs than surrounds other types of medication; probably because the illnesses for which they are prescribed even today still carry a certain stigma. We were able to illustrate this in a recent report on the safety of echinacea during pregnancy where 94% of the women in the study perceived the herb to be safe for use during pregnancy even though not a single study attested to its safety.[5]

Sudden discontinuation of antidepressants can cause patients to experience discontinuation symptoms or reemergence of the primary psychiatric disorder.[6] (The term *discontinuation* is preferred over *withdrawal* because withdrawal implies addiction or dependence.)

Antidepressants have an extremely low risk of abuse; they are not considered addictive agents.[7] Symptoms of discontinuation can include general somatic, gastrointestinal, affective, and sleep disturbances that tend to occur abruptly within days to weeks of stopping or reducing the dose. Reemergence of depression occurs more gradually.[8] Reinstitution of antidepressants mitigates the symptoms of discontinuation within a day, but it might take several weeks for a beneficial effect on depression to be felt.[9]

Although benzodiazepines can be abused, most patients do not abuse them.[10] Benzodiazepine dependence is well documented, however, and is characterized by loss of control over use of the drug, escalation of the dose, and much time spent acquiring and using the drug or recovering from its effects.[11] Patients physically dependent on benzodiazepines, whether they meet Diagnostic and Statistical Manual for Mental Disorders- Fourth Edition criteria for *abuse* or *dependence*, might experience symptoms following abrupt discontinuation.[12] Symptoms can last for weeks or months and can occur when even therapeutic doses are stopped suddenly. Patients report excessive anxiety, palpitations, insomnia, labile mood, and restlessness and can suffer from perceptual disturbances, primarily of vision and hearing. Seizures, psychosis, and delirium can also occur.[13,14]

We recently published a study documenting the adverse effects of 36 women who called the Motherisk Program after abruptly discontinuing either antidepressants or benzodiazepines (28 had discontinued the medications on the advice of their physicians). Before becoming pregnant, these women had been functioning well with their depression well controlled. They stopped the medication only because they feared it would harm their babies. All the women suffered abrupt discontinuation syndrome; 11 subsequently reported suicidal thoughts;

and 4 were later hospitalized. One of the remaining women had a therapeutic abortion, and one substituted alcohol for a benzodiazepine. After Motherisk's reassuring counseling, two thirds restarted their medication within several days. All babies born to mothers who restarted medication were normal and healthy.[15] Physicians should ensure that pregnant women with psychiatric disorders receive evidence-based information that balances the benefits of treatment against unproven adverse effects on unborn babies.

REFERENCES

1. Ceizel A. Lack of evidence of teratogenicity of benzodiazepine drugs in Hungary. *Reprod Toxicol* 1987;1:183–188.
2. Pastusak A, Schick-Boschetto B, Zuber C, et al. Pregnancy outcome following first trimester exposure to fluoxetine. *JAMA* 1993;269:2246–2248.
3. Kulin N, Pastusak A, Sage S, et al. Pregnancy outcome following maternal use of the new selective serotonin reuptake inhibitors: a prospective controlled multicentre study. *JAMA* 1998;279:609–610.
4. Nulman I, Rovet J, Stewart D, et al. Neurodevelopment of children exposed in utero to antidepressant drugs. *N Engl J Med* 1997;336:258–262.
5. Gallo M, Sarkar M, Au A, et al. The safety of echinacea in pregnancy: a prospective controlled study. *Arch Intern Med* 2000;160(20):3141–3143.
6. Rosenbaum JF, Fava M, Hoog SL, et al. Selective serotonin reuptake inhibitor discontinuation syndrome: a randomised clinical trial. *Biol Psychiatry* 1998;44(2):77–87.
7. Lejoyeux M. Dependence on antidepressive agents: an authentic addiction? *Encephale* 1995;21(1):63–65.
8. Kaplan EM. Antidepressant non compliance as a factor in the discontinuation syndrome. *J Clin Psych* 1997;58(Suppl. 7):31–35.
9. Dominguez RA, Goodnict PJ. Adverse events after abrupt discontinuation of paroxetine. *Pharmacotherapy* 1995;15(6):778–780.
10. Rickels K, Schweitzer E, Case WG, et al. Long term therapeutic use of benzodiazepines: effects of abrupt discontinuation. *Arch Gen Psychiatry* 1990;47(10):899–907.
11. Rickels K, Case WG, Schweitzer E, et al. Benzodiazepine dependence: management of discontinuation. *Psychopharmacol Bull* 1990;26(1): 63–68.
12. Turkington D, Gill P. Mania induced by lorazepam withdrawal: two case reports. *J Affect Dis* 1989;17(1):93–95.
13. Haque W, Watson DJ, Bryant SG. Death following suspected alprazolam withdrawal. A case report. *Tex Med* 1990;86(1):44–47.
14. Terao T, Tani Y. Two cases of psychotic state following normal dose benzodiazepine withdrawal. Sangyo Ika Daigaku Zasshi 1988;10(3):337–340.
15. Einarson A, Selby P, Koren G. Abrupt discontinuation of psychotropic drugs during pregnancy due to fears of teratogenic risk and the impact of counseling. *J Psychiatry Neurosci* 2001;26(1):44–48.

RISKS OF UNTREATED DEPRESSION DURING PREGNANCY

Adrienne Einarson, RN
Gideon Koren, MD, FRCPC

QUESTION

One of my patients who was taking an antidepressant for major depression is now pregnant and does not wish to take it any more. I believe she needs to continue her medication. She, however, is adamant about stopping it because she believes it would put her baby at risk. Is there evidence that not treating depression during pregnancy puts babies at risk?

Answer

A growing body of literature investigating the effects of not treating depression on mother and developing fetus suggests that untreated depression is associated with adverse fetal outcomes and a higher risk of maternal morbidity, including suicide ideation and attempts, and postpartum depression.

It is well known that women of childbearing age often suffer from major depression, which is most prevalent among people between 25 and 44 years old.[1] Estimates of lifetime risk in community-derived samples of pregnant women vary between 10% and 25%.[1-3] Although commonly used antidepressants have been shown to be safe during pregnancy,[4] women sometimes decide to discontinue these drugs when pregnancy is diagnosed out of fear of harming their babies.[5]

The literature examining risk of untreated depression during pregnancy suggests that psychopathologic symptoms during pregnancy have physiologic consequences for fetuses.[6] It has also been postulated that depression results in hazardous behaviors that can indirectly affect obstetric outcomes.

RISKY BEHAVIOR

Studies have found that mental illness can affect a mother's functional status and her ability to obtain prenatal care and avoid dangerous behavior. Mental illness can also affect decision-making capacities by causing cognitive distortions, and, because of this, it has been associated with poor attendance at antenatal clinics and malnutrition (which could lead to low birth weight babies).[7]

Depressed women are more likely to smoke and to use alcohol or other substances, which might compromise pregnancy. Depressed women can show deteriorating social function, emotional withdrawal, and excessive concern about their future ability to parent. They report excessive worry about pregnancy, are less likely to attend regular obstetric visits, and do not comply with prenatal advice. They take prenatal vitamins less often than nondepressed women and know less about the benefits of folic acid.[2,3,8] These behaviors all predict poor pregnancy outcome.

Severe depression also carries the risk of self-injurious, psychotic, impulsive, and harmful behaviors that can affect pregnancy. When patients refuse treatment, physicians should monitor patients for crises, such as suicide attempts, deteriorating social function, psychosis, and inability to comply with obstetric advice.[1]

LINKS TO ADVERSE OUTCOMES

Untreated depression during pregnancy has been linked to other adverse outcomes, such as spontaneous abortion,[9,10] increased uterine artery resistance,[11] small head circumference, low ApGAR scores, need for special neonatal care, neonatal growth retardation, preterm delivery, and babies with high cortisol levels at birth.[1,2,6–8,12–15] Studies also suggest that pregnant women who are depressed require more operative deliveries and report labor as more painful, which means they require more epidural analgesia. Gestational hypertension and subsequent preeclampsia has also been linked to untreated depression during pregnancy. Psychopathology during pregnancy is thought to affect the uterine environment and, therefore, could have an effect on fetal outcome. Current theories suggest that depression increases excretion of vasoactive hormones in the mother, and these hormones then mediate birth outcome. More research is needed to find out the exact mechanism.[7]

It is also evident that the risks of untreated depression do not end with birth. Women with untreated antenatal depression are also at increased risk of postpartum depression.[16] Studies have shown that these women are less capable of carrying out maternal duties and of bonding with their children.[17]

One study found elevated risk of preterm delivery (<37 weeks), low birth weight (<2500 g), and small for gestational age (<10th percentile) babies in women with Beck Depression Inventory (BDI) scores of 21 or more who were not receiving treatment.[15] Prenatal stress and depression have also been significantly associated with lower infant birth weight and younger gestational age at birth.[18,19] A recent study of lower social class women found that depression was associated with restricted fetal growth and small for gestational age babies.[20] There is also a clear association between increased hypothalamic, pituitary, and placental hormones in depressed mothers and the occurrence of preterm labour.[21]

Studies have investigated the link between depression and preeclampsia. Strenuous work, depression, and anxiety might increase risk of this condition, but the stress of daily living has not been associated with it. In Finland, 623 nulliparous women at low risk of preeclampsia all had healthy first trimesters and were then tested for depression and anxiety at about 12 weeks' gestation. Depression (odds ratio 2.5, 95% confidence interval 1.2 to 5.3) and anxiety were both associated with increased risk of preeclampsia.[6]

CONCLUSION

A growing body of literature suggests that the risk of adverse effects of untreated depression in pregnancy is high. Because selective serotonin reuptake inhibitors have been shown to be safe during pregnancy, the risk-benefit ratio is quite clear.

REFERENCES

1. Wisner KL, Zarin DA, Holmboe ES, et al. Risk-benefit decision making for treatment of depression during pregnancy. *Am J Psychiatry* 2000; 157(12):1933–1940.
2. Nonacs R, Cohen LS. Depression during pregnancy: diagnosis and treatment options. *J Clin Psychiatry* 2002;63(7):24–30.
3. Burt VK, Stein K. Epidemiology of depression throughout the female life cycle. *J Clin Psychiatry* 2002;63(Suppl. 7):9–15.

4. Addis A, Koren G. Safety of fluoxetine during the first trimester of pregnancy: a meta-analytical review of epidemiological studies. *Psychol Med* 2000;30(1):89–94.

5. Einarson A, Selby P, Koren G. Abrupt discontinuation of psychotropic drugs during pregnancy: fear of teratogenic risk and impact of counselling. *J Psychiatry Neurosci* 2001;26(1):44–48.

6. Kurki T, Hiilesmaa V, Raitasalo R, et al. Depression and anxiety in early pregnancy and risk for preeclampsia. *Obstet Gynecol* 2000;95(4):487–490.

7. Evans J, Heron J, Francomb H, et al. Cohort study of depressed mood during pregnancy and after childbirth. *BMJ* 2001;323(7307):257–260.

8. Zuckerman B, Amaro H, Bauchner H, et al. Depressive symptoms during pregnancy: relationship to poor health behaviors. *Am J Obstet Gynecol* 1989;160(5 Pt. 1):1107–1111.

9. Arck PC. Pregnancy loss. *Am J Reprod Immunol* 2001;45:303–309.

10. Sugiura-Ogasawara M, Furukawa TA, Nakano Y, et al. Depression as a potential causal factor in subsequent miscarriage in recurrent spontaneous aborters. *Hum Reprod* 2002;17(10):2580–2584.

11. Teixeira JM, Fisk NM, Glover V. Association between maternal anxiety in pregnancy and increased uterine artery resistance index: cohort based study. *BMJ* 1999;318(7177):153–157.

12. Chung TK, Lau TK, Yip AS, et al. Antepartum depressive symptomatology is associated with adverse obstetric and neonatal outcomes. *Psychosom Med* 2001;63(5):830–834.

13. Ashman SB, Dawson G, Panagiotides H, et al. Stress hormone levels of children of depressed mothers. *Dev Psychopathol* 2002;14(2):333–349.

14. Orr ST, Miller CA. Maternal depressive symptoms and the risk of poor pregnancy outcome. Review of the literature and preliminary findings. *Epidemiol Rev* 1995;17(1):165–171.

15. Steer RA, Scholl TO, Hediger ML, et al. Self-reported depression and negative pregnancy outcomes. *J Clin Epidemiol* 1992;45(10):1093–1099.

16. Marcus SM, Flynn HA, Blow FC, et al. J Womens Health. In press.

17. Bosquet M, Egeland B. Associations among maternal depressive symptomatology, state of mind and parent and child behaviors: implications for attachment-based interventions. *Attach Hum Dev* 2001;3(2):173–199.

18. Wadhwa PD, Sandman CA, Porto M, et al. The association between prenatal stress and infant birth weight and gestational age at birth: a prospective investigation. *Am J Obstet Gynecol* 1993;169:858–865.

19. Hostetter A, Szsjjmel A. Dose of selective serotonin uptake inhibitors across pregnancy: clinical implications. *Depress Anxiety* 2000;11(2):51–57.

20. Hoffman S, Hatch MC. Depressive symptomatology during pregnancy: evidence for an association with decreased fetal growth in pregnancies of lower social class women. *Health Psychol* 2000;19(6):535–543.

21. Weinstock M. Alterations induced by gestational stress in brain morphology and behaviour of the offspring. *Prog Neurobiol* 2001;65(5):427–451.

TAKING ANTIDEPRESSANTS DURING LATE PREGNANCY—HOW SHOULD WE ADVISE WOMEN?

Sanjog Kalra, MSc
Adrienne Einarson, RN
Gideon Koren MD, FRCPC

QUESTION

In light of recent negative media attention to antidepressant use during late pregnancy, several of my patients have either discontinued or are considering discontinuing their antidepressant medications. How can I best counsel these patients on taking antidepressants during late pregnancy?

Answer

Antidepressant use during the third trimester has been associated occasionally with a transient neonatal withdrawal-like syndrome characterized by jitteriness, self-limiting respiratory difficulties, and problems with feeding. When counseling patients, the risk of these adverse effects must be weighed against the risks associated with untreated depression during late pregnancy. Abrupt discontinuation of psychotropic medications has been associated with both physical (e.g., withdrawal) and psychological (e.g., suicidal thoughts) symptoms.

The World Health Organization has identified depression as a leading cause of morbidity in the 21st century.[1] Depression is expected to become the second largest worldwide cause of disease burden by 2020.[2] Given that depression is about three times more common in women than in men and that its peak prevalence occurs between 25 and 44 years of age,[3] many women will require treatment for depression while pregnant.

A growing body of evidence attests to the fetal safety of antidepressants commonly used during pregnancy. Various prospective controlled studies have examined the physical and neurodevelopmental safety of tricyclic antidepressants, as well as selective serotonin reuptake inhibitor (SSRI) and selective norepinephrine reuptake inhibitor (SNRI) medications during the first trimester and throughout pregnancy.[4]

Some studies have described a poor neonatal adaptation syndrome in newborns whose mothers had been taking tricyclic, SSRI, or SNRI antidepressants near term.[5-9] Although not yet clearly defined, the most common adverse effects associated with this syndrome are transient, mostly self-limiting, jitteriness; grasping muscle weakness; and respiratory difficulties that sometimes require use of a ventilator.[6] Currently, Motherisk recommends that infants born to mothers taking antidepressants during late pregnancy be closely monitored for longer than the typical 24 to 48 hours after birth.

Health Canada recently published an advisory suggesting that women and their physicians consider slowly decreasing the dose of these medications during late pregnancy.[10] After this advisory appeared in the media, the Motherisk Program received many calls from concerned women and their health care providers wondering whether it was safe to use antidepressants during late pregnancy. Some women reported having abruptly discontinued their antidepressant medications.[11]

In assessing the risks and benefits of using antidepressants during late pregnancy, physicians need to consider the risks of discontinuing these medications near term and the risks of untreated depression during the third trimester. Neonatal risks appear to be limited to development of poor neonatal adaptability in 10% to 30% of babies.[5-9]

Untreated depression during pregnancy has been associated with miscarriage, perinatal complications, increased risk of preeclampsia, low neonatal Apgar scores, and increased admissions to neonatal intensive care units.[12] The most serious maternal ramification of untreated depression during pregnancy is an increased risk of postpartum depression, which can have tragic consequences.[13]

Among pregnant women, abrupt discontinuation of antidepressants has been associated with withdrawal symptoms, including nausea and vomiting, diarrhea, sweating, anxiety and panic attacks, mood swings, and suicidal thoughts.[14] Abrupt discontinuation of medications could also allow the primary psychiatric condition to resurface.[15]

The adverse effects on mothers and babies of untreated depression during pregnancy combined with the known (serious) risks associated with abrupt discontinuation of psychotropic medications appear to outweigh the risk of transient poor neonatal adaptation in only a very few neonates exposed to antidepressants during the third trimester.

After consultation with their physicians, women who decide to discontinue or taper their doses of antidepressants should do so as gradually as possible over several weeks. Women's moods and fetal well-being should be closely monitored during this period, especially after delivery.

REFERENCES

1. Buist A. Managing depression in pregnancy. *Aust Fam Physician* 2000; 29(7):663–667.
2. Murray CJ, Lopez AD. Evidence-based health policy lessons from the Global Burden of Disease Study. *Science* 1996;274(5288):740–743.
3. Weissman MM, Bland R, Joyce PR, et al. Sex differences in rates of depression: cross-national perspectives. *J Affect Disord* 1993;29(2–3):77–84.
4. Kalra SB, Sarkar M, Einarson A. Safety of antidepressants in pregnancy. *Expert Opin Drug Saf* 2005;4(2):273–284.
5. Chambers CD, Johnson KA, Dick LM, et al. Birth outcomes in pregnant women taking fluoxetine. *N Engl J Med* 1996;335(14):1010–1015. Comments in *N Engl J Med* 1996;335(14):1056–1058. *N Engl J Med* 1997;336(12):872–873,author reply 873.
6. Costei AM, Kozer E, Ho T, et al. Perinatal outcome following third trimester exposure to paroxetine. *Arch Pediatr Adolesc Med* 2002; 156(11):1129–1132.
7. Hendrick V, Smith LM, Suri R, et al. Birth outcomes after prenatal exposure to antidepressant medication. *Am J Obstet Gynecol* 2003;188(3): 812–815.
8. Oberlander TF, Misri S, Fitzgerald CE, et al. Pharmacologic factors associated with transient neonatal symptoms following prenatal psychotropic medication exposure. *J Clin Psychiatry* 2004;65(2):230–237.
9. Kallen B. Neonate characteristics after maternal use of antidepressants in late pregnancy. *Arch Pediatr Adolesc Med* 2004;158(4):312–316.
10. Health Canada advises of potential adverse effects of SSRIs and other antidepressants on newborns [advisory]. Health Canada Online 2004(Aug 9); 2004–2044. Available from http://www.hc-sc.gc.ca/english/protection/warnings/2004/2004_44.htm. Accessed 2005 July 12.
11. Einarson A, Schachtschneider AM, Halil R, et al. SSRI's and other antidepressant use during pregnancy and potential neonatal adverse effects. Impact of a public health advisory and subsequent reports in the news media. *BMC Pregnancy and Childbirth* 2005;5:11.
12. Bonari L, Pinto N, Ahn E, et al. Perinatal risks of untreated depression during pregnancy. *Can J Psychiatry* 2004;49(11):726–735.

13. Beck CT. Revision of the Postpartum Depression Predictors Inventory. *J Obstet Gynecol Neonatal Nurs* 2002;31(4):394–402.
14. Einarson A, Selby P, Koren G. Abrupt discontinuation of psychotropic drugs during pregnancy: fear of teratogenic risk and impact of counselling. *J Psychiatry Neurosci* 2001;26(1):44–48.
15. Rosenbaum JF, Zajecka J. Clinical management of antidepressant discontinuation. *J Clin Psychiatry* 1997;58(Suppl. 7):37–40.

TAKING ST. JOHN'S WORT DURING PREGNANCY

Ran D. Goldman, MD
Gideon Koren, MD, FRCPC

QUESTION

A 23-year-old patient of mine has been taking St. John's wort for postpartum depression for about 2 years. She is now planning her second pregnancy. Is she or her fetus at risk if she continues to take the herbal therapy?

Answer

Despite the widespread availability and use of St. John's wort and extensive research on the herb, there are almost no data on reproductive safety. At this stage, therefore, St. John's wort cannot be recommended as safe therapy during pregnancy.

In North America, St. John's wort is a dietary supplement; in 1998, total retail sales in the United States totaled $140 million.[1-2] St. John's wort contains at least 10 different active substances; hypericin is considered the most active ingredient.[3] The herbal extract displays the pharmacologic qualities of several antidepressants by inhibiting the synaptic reuptake of serotonin, dopamine, and noradrenaline.[4]

RESULTS OF STUDIES

Linde and Mulrow[5] published a meta-analysis that included 2291 patients with *neurotic depression* or *mild to moderately severe depressive disorders* from 27 trials. The reviewers concluded that the evidence indicated St. John's wort was more effective than placebo for short-term treatment of mild-to-moderate depressive disorders. Although unable to conclude that St. John's wort was better treatment than other antidepressants, they stated that it seemed comparable to maprotiline, imipramine, and amitriptyline.

In a recent double-blind, randomized placebo-controlled trial, the efficacy and safety of a well characterized Hypericum perforatum preparation was compared with placebo or sertraline for 8 weeks. Participants were adult outpatients with major depression. Neither St. John's wort nor sertraline was significantly better than placebo.[6] St. John's wort is well tolerated and is perceived as safer than most antidepressants prescribed in Canada. It can, however, have adverse effects[5,7-9] and interact with other drugs.[2] About 2% to 26% of patients using St. John's wort report side effects that include nausea and restlessness (most common), delayed hypersensitivity, dizziness, dry mouth, and constipation. Photodermatitis is a rare, but well recognized, adverse effect. St. John's wort's ability to induce the cytochrome P-4503A metabolizing enzyme might put transplant patients receiving cyclosporine at risk of graft rejection.

St. John's wort can be found at most pharmacies, natural food stores, and some grocery stores in Canada, and hence it is widely available to women of childbearing age. Whether recommended by a family physician or taken without recommendation, St. John's wort could be harmful before pregnancy is diagnosed or during pregnancy.

Responses from a randomly selected group of Canadian physicians, medical students, naturopaths, and naturopathic students to a detailed questionnaire (242 respondents; 38% response rate) showed that St. John's wort was the second most popular complementary medicine recommended by both medical doctors and naturopaths (*Echinacea* was first). Although only one physician recommended a herbal product to a pregnant patient, as many as 49% of the naturopaths felt comfortable recommending herbal products to pregnant women.[9] To date, three animal studies have addressed use of St. John's wort during the perinatal period. No reproductive toxic effects were found in rats or dogs with oral doses of 900 and 2700 mg/kg.[10] When a group of female mice receiving Hypericum from 2 weeks before conception and throughout gestation was compared with a group of female mice receiving placebo, one study[11] found that mouse offspring in both groups were similar in gestational age at delivery, litter size, perinatal outcome, body weight, body length, and head circumference growth through adulthood. Moreover, no differences were found in reaching physical milestones, in reproductive capability, or in growth and development of second-generation offspring. A similar study found lower birth weights among male offspring in the St. John's wort group, but no long-term differences in early developmental tasks, locomotor activity, or exploratory behaviour throughout development.[12]

SELF-TREATMENT

Only two cases of women treating themselves with St. John's wort during pregnancy are reported in the literature.[13] In one case, where follow up was available, a woman took the herb from 24 weeks gestation until delivery. Her neonate was reported to have normal results of physical examination and behavioral assessment during the first month of life. A recent controlled study completed by Motherisk has failed to show increased teratogenic risk with St. John's Wort. (Morett M. personal).

Not enough data are available to conclude that St. John's wort is safe for pregnant women or fetuses. Much more preclinical and clinical data must be accumulated before the herb can safely be regulated as an adjunct or alternative treatment to the antidepressant drugs currently prescribed for pregnant women.

REFERENCES

1. Muller WE, Kasper S. Clinically used antidepressant drugs. *Pharmacopsychiatry* 1997;30(Suppl. 2):71.
2. Ernst E. The risk-benefit profile of commonly used herbal therapies: ginkgo, St. John's wort, ginseng, echinacea, saw palmetto, and kava. *Ann Intern Med* 2002;136:42–53. 1982;142:85–89.
3. Muller WE, Singer A, Wonnemann M. Hyperforin represents the neurotransmitter reuptake inhibiting constituent of Hypericum extract. *Pharmacopsychiatry* 1998;31(Suppl. 1):16–21.
4. Nathan P. The experimental and clinical pharmacology of St. John's wort (Hypericum perforatum L). *Mol Psychiatry* 1999;4:333–338.
5. Linde K, Mulrow CD. St. John's wort for depression. *Cochrane Database Syst Rev* 2000;CD000448.
6. Hypericum Depression Trial Study Group. Effect of Hypericum perforatum (St. John's wort) in major depressive disorders: a randomized controlled trial. *JAMA* 2002;287:1807–1814.
7. Woelk H, Burkard G, Grunwald J. Benefits and risks of the Hypericum extract LI 160: drug-monitoring study with 3250 patients. *J Geriatr Psychiatry Neurol* 1994;7(Suppl. 1):S34–S38.
8. Schrader E, Meier B, Brattstrom A. Hepericum treatment of mild-moderate depression in a placebo-controlled study. *Hum Psychopharmacol* 1998;13:163–169.

9. Einarson A, Lawrimore T, Brand P, et al. Attitudes and practices of physicians and naturopaths toward herbal products, including use during pregnancy and lactation. *Can J Clin Pharmacol* 2000;7:45–49.

10. Upton R, Graffa WE, Buneing D, et al. St. John's wort monograph. *Am Herbal Pharmacopoeia* 1997:1–32.

11. Rayburn WF, Gonzalez CL, Christensen HD, et al. Effect of prenatally administered Hypericum (St. John's wort) on growth and physical maturation of mouse offspring. *Am J Obstet Gynecol* 2001;184:191–195.

12. Rayburn WF, Christensen HD, Gonzalez CL. Effect of antenatal exposure to St. John's wort (Hypericum) on neurobehavior of developing mice. *Am J Obstet Gynecol* 2000;183:1225–1231.

13. Grush LR, Nierenberg A, Keefe B, et al. St. John's wort during pregnancy. *JAMA* 1998;280:1566.

CHAPTER 44

TRIMETHOPRIM-SULFONAMIDE COMBINATION THERAPY IN EARLY PREGNANCY

Adrienne Einarson, RN
Samar R. Shuhaiber, MSc
Gideon Koren, MD, FRCPC

QUESTION

One of my patients presented with bacteriuria early in her pregnancy. Urine culture was positive for Escherichia coli. I would like to prescribe a trimethoprim-sulfamethoxazole combination because it worked well for her in the past. What is known about the safety of this medication during early pregnancy?

Answer

Evidence-based studies report an association between trimethoprim-sulfonamide (TMP-SMX) combinations in early pregnancy and several major malformations, such as neural tube defects and cardiovascular defects. If clinically possible, physicians are advised to use alternative antimicrobial medications for treatment of urinary tract infections (UTIs) during early pregnancy.

UTIs are common among pregnant women. Untreated UTIs can progress to acute pyelonephritis and other ascending infections. There is a link between untreated genitourinary infections in pregnancy and premature labor that could be explained by the cytokines and prostaglandins released by microorganisms.[1] In the United States, 40% of preterm deliveries are thought to be the result of infections.[1] The goal of treating genitourinary infections during pregnancy is to administer appropriate antimicrobial medications to eradicate susceptible infection and to protect the developing fetus.

TMP-SMX combinations are used to treat a variety of infections caused by Gram-positive and Gram-negative bacteria. TMP-SMX combinations have been widely indicated for acute and uncomplicated UTIs in women. Several European and American surveys on antibiotic use indicate that trimethoprim alone or TMP-SMX combinations are among the first-line treatments for UTIs.[2,3] Both trimethoprim and sulfonamide antibiotics inhibit nucleic acid synthesis by interfering with bacterial production of folic acid. Although trimethoprim and sulfonamide are highly specific to bacteria, several recent studies have suggested that folic acid antagonists taken during pregnancy are associated with increased risk of neural tube defects (NTDs) and other congenital defects.

A recent case-control study of birth defects in the United States and Canada reported that women giving birth to children with NTDs had an odds ratio (OR) of 2.8 (95% confidence interval [CI] 1.7–4.6) of having been exposed to TMP-SMX during early pregnancy compared with women giving birth to healthy children.[4]

Another case-control study of birth defects in Hungary examined the safety of TMP-SMX combinations during pregnancy.[5] A higher rate of trimethoprim-sulfamethazine and TMP-SMX use was reported among mothers of children with cardiovascular and multiple birth defects (OR 6.4, 95% CI 2.0–20.3 and OR 2.1, 95% CI 1.4–3.3, respectively).

Treatment with TMP-SMX during the first month of pregnancy was associated with a significant increase in NTDs (OR 4.3, 95% CI 2.1–8.6). The study also reported that, when women receiving therapy with TMP-SMX were taking additional folic acid supplementation of 6 mg/day, fewer of them had babies with birth defects (OR 1.87, 95% CI 1.25–2.77).

The Michigan Medicaid surveillance study found that, among 2296 children exposed to TMP-SMX combinations in utero, 37 (1.6%) babies developed cardiovascular defects (only 23 cardiac defects were expected).[6] Overall, there were 126 (5.5%) birth defects observed in this study (only 98 were expected). Other confounding factors, such as maternal age, disease, and other drug use, were not evaluated. Another large retrospective study, the Collaborative Perinatal Project, monitored 1455 mother-child pairs exposed to sulfonamides during the first trimester and found no association with any particular group of birth defects.[7]

In theory, sulfonamides should also be avoided after 32 weeks' gestation because of their associated toxicity in newborns. Sulfonamides could displace bilirubin from albumin-binding sites and could cause severe jaundice leading to kernicterus.[8] Practical evidence of this risk, however, is sparse. Acute hemolytic anemia is another complication that could occur in newborns with glucose-6-phosphate dehydrogenase deficiency.[9]

In summary, trimethoprim alone or TMP-SMX combinations should be avoided if possible during the first trimester of pregnancy. Whenever clinically feasible, alternative antibiotics should be considered for treatment of UTIs. Other classes of antibiotics, such as penicillins, cephalosporins, nitrofurantoin, and macrolides, are relatively safe choices for treating bacterial infections during pregnancy.[10] If TMP-SMX is clinically required during the first month of pregnancy, a higher dose of folic acid (4 mg/day) should be given to prevent NTDs.

REFERENCES

1. Cram L, Zapata MI, Toy E, et al. Genitourinary infections and their association with preterm labour. *Am Fam Physician* 2002;65(2):241–248.
2. Naber KG. Survey on antibiotic usage in the treatment of urinary tract infections. *J Antimicrob Chemother* 2000;46(Suppl. 1):49–52.
3. Huang E, Stafford RS. National patterns in the treatment of urinary tract infections in women by ambulatory care physicians. *Arch Intern Med* 2002;162(1):41–47.
4. Hernandez-Diaz S, Werler MM, Walker AM, et al. Neural tube defects in relation to use of folic acid antagonists during pregnancy. *Am J Epidemiol* 2001;153(10):961–968.
5. Czeisel A, Rockenbaer M, et al. The teratogenic risk of trimethoprim-sulfonamides: a population based case-control study. *Reprod Toxicol* 2001; 15:637–646.
6. Briggs G. Drugs in pregnancy and lactation 7th ed, Lippincott Williams & Wilkins; 2005.
7. Heinonen OP, Slone D, Shapiro S. *Birth Defects and Drugs in Pregnancy.* Littleton, Md: Publishing Sciences Group; 1977.
8. Dunn PM. The possible relationship between the maternal administration of sulphamethoxypyridazine and hyperbilirubinaemia in the newborn. *J Obstet Gynaecol Br Commonw* 1964;71:128–131.
9. Perkins RP. Hydrops fetalis and stillbirth in a male glucose-6-phosphate dehydrogenase-deficient fetus possibly due to maternal ingestion of sulfisoxazole. *Am J Obstet Gynecol* 1971;111:379–381.
10. Einarson A, Shuhaiber S, Koren G. Effects of antibacterials on the unborn child. *Paediatr drugs* 2001;3(11):803–816.

CHAPTER 45

INFLUENZA VACCINATION DURING PREGNANCY

Ran D. Goldman, MD
Gideon Koren, MD, FRCPC

QUESTION

A 27-year-old patient of mine recently learned she is pregnant. She took the influenza vaccine offered at work when she was 7 weeks pregnant. Is her fetus at risk of malformations?

Answer

No evidence indicates that killed-influenza vaccine is teratogenic, even if given during the first trimester. Since 1996, Health Canada's Centre for Disease Control and Prevention has recommended that pregnant women in their second and third trimesters be vaccinated. This should not be interpreted as evidence that the vaccine is teratogenic in the first trimester because such evidence does not exist.

Influenza is an acute respiratory illness brought on by virus types A or B. The disease causes rapid onset of fever, myalgia, malaise, sore throat, and nonproductive cough. The incubation period is 1 to 3 days, and the virus can undergo transition up to 7 days after the onset of illness. Complications, such as pneumonia, exacerbation of chronic illness, and even death, have been reported in North America during influenza epidemics.[1,2]

Influenza vaccine consists of purified virus proteins. Because the virus changes its antigenic profile almost every year, researchers predict the influenza antigenicity of the three most common strains of the virus, and the vaccine is prepared based on that. That is why annual immunization is needed.

The influenza vaccine is safe, effective, and cost-effective,[3] and could prevent illness in 70% to 90% of healthy people younger than 65 years.[4] The government of Ontario has recently decided to immunize all high-risk populations.[5] Adverse effects of the vaccine include a mild form of influenza and allergic reactions in people with allergy to eggs (the vaccine is manufactured using an egg substrate). Severe adverse effects are rare; Guillain-Barré syndrome occurs in about one of every million people vaccinated.[6]

Pregnant women face an increased risk of morbidity and stillbirth if they get influenza, as was shown in a few outbreaks in the 1910s and 1950s.[7] Women with medical conditions that increase their risk of complications from influenza, such as chronic pulmonary or cardiac illness during the year before conception,[8] should be vaccinated.[9,10] In 1996, Health Canada's Centre for Disease Control and Prevention added pregnant women in their second and third trimesters to the list of high-risk populations they recommended be vaccinated (http://www.cdc.gov/ncidod/diseases/flu/fluvac.htm).[11,12]

STUDIES

One case report described a baby girl born with cerebral malformations characterized by developmental arrest late in the first trimester of gestation.[13] Her mother had received influenza vaccine 6 weeks after conception and had been ill for 2 weeks following that. The authors could not conclude whether the vaccine was teratogenic or whether the vaccination and malformations appeared coincidentally.

Two studies prospectively investigated the effects of the vaccine on maternal health and outcomes of pregnancy and on the health of the infants at 2 months old. Sumaya and Gibbs[14] reported on a study of 56 women who received inactivated influenza A/New Jersey/76 virus vaccine during their second and third trimesters. No severe immediate reactions or increased fetal complications associated with administration of the vaccine were observed. Deinard and Ogburn[15] reported the outcomes of the pregnancies of 189 women who received the same vaccine. Their longitudinal, prospective study found no association between immunization and maternal, perinatal, or infant complications. Study women were compared with 517 pregnant women who did not receive the vaccine. No teratogenicity was observed, and the two groups of infants were similar in physical and neurologic development at birth and at 8 weeks old.

INFLUENZA ANTIGENS

Because maternal influenza antigens can cross the placenta,[16] vaccinating pregnant women could provide newborns with high antibody titres to the influenza virus that would protect them until self-immunization is likely to be protective.[17] Sumaya and Gibbs[14] reported that the 56 women in their study responded to the vaccine the same way nonpregnant adults did. At delivery, almost half of 40 maternal-fetal pairs had notable antibody titre levels in neonatal cord serum. At 6 months old, only one infant had a detectable antibody level. The authors recommended administration of a more potent influenza vaccine.[14]

CONCLUSION

The risk of maternal and fetal morbidity and mortality from influenza seems to be greater than the theoretical risk of adverse effects on pregnancy outcome posed by the killed virus vaccine. There is no evidence that the vaccine is teratogenic, even if it is given during the first trimester.

REFERENCES

1. Barker WH. Excess pneumonia and influenza associated hospitalization during influenza epidemics in the United States, 1970-78. Am J Public Health 1986;76:761–765.
2. Barker WH, Mullooly JP. Pneumonia and influenza deaths during epidemics: implications for prevention. Arch Intern Med 1982;142:85–89.
3. Campbell DS, Rumley MH. Cost-effectiveness of the influenza vaccine in healthy, working-age populations. J Occup Environ Med 1997;39:408–414.
4. Hall CB, Douglas RG Jr, Geiman JM. Respiratory syncytial virus infections in infants: quantitation and duration of shedding. J Pediatr 1976;89:11–15.
5. Schabas RE. Mass influenza vaccination in Ontario: a sensible move. Can Med Assoc J 2001;164:36–37.
6. Lasky T, Terracciano GJ, Magder L, et al. The Guillain-Barre syndrome and the 1992–1993 and 1993–1994 influenza vaccines. N Engl J Med 1998;339:1797–1802.
7. Ramphal R, Donnelly WH, Small PA. Fatal influenzal pneumonia in pregnancy: failure to demonstrate transplacental transmission of influenza virus. Am J Obstet Gynecol 1980;138:347–348.
8. Sterner G, Grandien M, Enocksson E. Pregnant women with acute respiratory illness at term. Scand J Infect Dis Suppl 1990;71:19–26.

9. Philit F, Cordier JF. Therapeutic approaches of clinicians to influenza pandemic. *Eur J Epidemiol* 1994;10:491–492.

10. Prevention and control of influenza. *MMWR Morb Mortal Wkly Rep* 1988;37:361–364,369–373.

11. Prevention and control of influenza: recommendations of the Advisory Committee on Immunization Practices (ACIP). Centres for Disease Control and Prevention. *MMWR Morb Mortal Wkly Rep* 1996;45(RR-5): 1–24.

12. Bridges CB, Fukuda K, Cox NJ, et al. Prevention and control of influenza. Recommendations of the Advisory Committee on Immunization Practices (ACIP). *MMWR Morb Mortal Wkly Rep* 2001;50(RR-4):1–44.

13. Sarnat HB, Rybak G, Kotagal S, et al. Cerebral embryopathy in late first trimester: possible association with swine influenza vaccine. *Teratology* 1979;20:93–99.

14. Sumaya CV, Gibbs RS. Immunization of pregnant women with influenza A/New Jersey/76 virus vaccine: reactogenicity and immunogenicity in mother and infant. *J Infect Dis* 1979;140:141–146.

15. Deinard AS, Ogburn P Jr. A/NJ/8/76 influenza vaccination program: effects on maternal health and pregnancy outcome. *Am J Obstet Gynecol* 1981;140:240–245.

16. Yawn DH, Pyeatte JC, Joseph JM, et al. Transplacental transfer of influenza virus. *JAMA* 1971;216:1022–1023.

17. Linder N, Ohel G. In utero vaccination. *Clin Perinatol* 1994;21: 663–674.

CHAPTER 46

ANTIRETROVIRAL TREATMENT OF MATERNAL HIV INFECTION

Alejandro A. Nava-Ocampo, MD
Gideon Koren, MD, FRCPC

QUESTION

One of my pregnant patients tested positive for human immunodeficiency virus (HIV). Will HIV therapy put her pregnancy outcome at risk?

Answer

The biggest risk is vertical transmission of HIV to her baby. She should be treated with combination therapy; triple therapy is required to reduce vertical transmission. Zidovudine (AZT) is not teratogenic in humans, but information on other antiretroviral drugs is incomplete.

Mother-to-child transmission of HIV can be reduced from 25% to less than 2% by appropriate antiretroviral therapy (ARV) and avoiding breastfeeding.[1] Use of ARV drugs during pregnancy might require dose adjustments because of the physiologic changes associated with pregnancy. The current consensus is that therapy should be initiated with three drugs, either a combination of two nucleoside analogue reverse transcriptase inhibitors (NARTI) and a protease inhibitor (PI) or a combination of two NARTIs and a non-nucleoside reverse transcriptase inhibitor (NNRTI).[1]

In a 10-year longitudinal epidemiologic study, vertical transmission of HIV was observed in 20% of women with HIV-1 infection who received no ARV treatment during pregnancy, in 10.4% who received AZT alone, in 3.8% who received combination therapy without PIs, and in 1.2% who received combination therapy with PIs.[2] These results are similar to results in other studies. These studies also found no increase in rates of preterm labor, low birth weight, low Apgar scores, or stillbirth in suboptimally treated women.[3,4]

FOUR CLINICAL SITUATIONS

In discussing HIV during pregnancy, four clinical situations should be considered.[3]

WOMEN WHO HAVE NOT RECEIVED ARV THERAPY

Regardless of antenatal virus load, an AZT chemoprophylaxis regimen, initiated after the first trimester, should be recommended to all pregnant women with HIV-1 infection.[2-5] A combination of AZT with an additional ARV drug is recommended for infected women whose HIV-1 Ribonucleic acid is more than 1000 copies/mL regardless of clinical or immunologic status.[6] Women in the first trimester can consider delaying initiation of therapy until after 10 to 12 weeks' gestation because the risks associated with various agents during organogenesis (the first 10 weeks of gestation) are largely unknown.[3,7] We know the extent to which AZT passes through the placenta, but we do not know if this transfer is similar for other ARV drugs.[1,8] If a woman does not receive AZT as a component of her antenatal ARV regimen, she should receive AZT therapy during the intrapartum period and her newborn should receive it also.[9-11]

WOMEN WHO HAVE RECEIVED ARV THERAPY DURING THE CURRENT PREGNANCY

These patients should continue therapy; AZT should be included as a component of the antenatal ARV regimen after the first trimester whenever possible, although this might not always be feasible.[12] Women receiving ARV therapy in whom pregnancy is recognized during the first trimester should be counseled regarding the benefits and risks of such therapy during this period. Continuation of therapy should be considered. If therapy is discontinued during the first trimester, all drugs should be stopped and reintroduced simultaneously to avoid development of drug resistance.[13] Regardless of antepartum ARV regimen, AZT is recommended during the intrapartum period and for newborns.[2,11]

WOMEN WHO ARE IN LABOR AND HAVE HAD NO PRIOR THERAPY

Two effective regimens have been documented. Intrapartum AZT intravenously followed by 6 weeks of AZT for the newborn, or oral AZT and lamivudine (3TC) during labor followed by 1 week of oral AZT or 3TC for the newborn[1,3,5,8,9,11,14–17] have been recommended. A single dose of nevirapine at onset of labor followed by a single dose of nevirapine for the newborn at 48 hours old has also been recommended.[7,12,13,18–21] The second regimen involves two doses of nevirapine combined with intrapartum AZT intravenously and 6 weeks of oral AZT for the newborn.[19–22] In the immediate postpartum period, women should have appropriate assessment (CD4+ count and HIV-1 RNA copy number) in order to plan continuation of therapy.

INFANTS BORN TO MOTHERS WHO HAVE RECEIVED NO ARV THERAPY DURING PREGNANCY OR THE INTRAPARTUM PERIOD

Between 7% and 40% of infants born to HIV-positive mothers become infected. The prognosis of these infants is poor; most develop early and rapidly progressive disease.[23] At 6 weeks, neonatal AZT should be offered to newborns. AZT therapy should be initiated as soon as possible after delivery, preferably within 6 to 12 hours of birth. Some clinicians use AZT in combination with other ARV drugs, particularly if a mother is suspected of having an AZT-resistant virus.[4,5,23] Efficacy for infants is currently unknown. In the immediate postpartum period, mother and infant should undergo diagnostic testing to tailor appropriate therapy.

TYPES OF ARV DRUGS

There are four different types of ARV drugs and only partial information on their fetal safety.

NUCLEOSIDE ANALOGUE REVERSE TRANSCRIPTASE INHIBITORS

AZT and 3TC are well tolerated during pregnancy.[16,24] Infants exposed in utero to AZT and followed up for approximately 6 years appeared similar to healthy controls.[25,26] No evidence indicates an increased rate of congenital abnormalities among infants born to women with antepartum exposure to AZT.[2,25,27]

The pharmacokinetics of 3TC are similar in pregnant women and nonpregnant women; no pharmacokinetic interactions with AZT have been reported.[14,16,17,24] Similarly, the pharmacokinetics of didanosine and stavudine are not affected by pregnancy.[24,27,28] Abacavir exhibits developmental toxicity and increased incidence of fetal anasarca and skeletal malformations in animals. Zalcitabine (ddC) appeared to be teratogenic (hydrocephalus) in rats.[27,29]

The NARTI drugs might induce mitochondrial dysfunction characterized by neuropathy, myopathy, cardiomyopathy, pancreatitis, hepatic steatosis, and lactic acidosis (the two latter might have a female preponderance).[30–32] These drugs occasionally produce a life-threatening syndrome of acute fatty liver of pregnancy and hemolysis, elevated liver enzymes, and low platelet count (the HELLP syndrome) during the third trimester of pregnancy.[32] Whether mitochondrial dysfunction affects fetuses is still debated; case reports suggest a positive association, but population-based studies refute that. Hepatic enzymes and electrolytes should be assessed more frequently during the last trimester, and any new symptoms should be evaluated thoroughly.

NONNUCLEOSIDE ANALOGUE REVERSE TRANSCRIPTASE INHIBITORS

Delavirdine is teratogenic in rats, but has not been evaluated in HIV-infected pregnant women. Efavirenz exhibits teratogenic effects in primates and should be avoided in pregnant women until more information is available. Severe, life-threatening and, in some cases, fatal hepatotoxicity, including cholestatic and fulminant hepatitis, hepatic necrosis, and hepatic failure, have been reported in HIV-infected patients receiving nevirapine in combination with other drugs for prophylaxis against nosocomial or sexual HIV exposure.[22,27,32]

Protease inhibitors Hyperglycemia and diabetes mellitus have been reported among patients taking PIs.[33,34] Limited data show almost 80% of women taking PIs developed one or more typical adverse effects, such as anemia, nausea, vomiting, aminotransferase elevation, and hyperglycemia.[27,31–34] Clinical trials on indinavir, ritonavir, nelfinavir, and saquinavir are ongoing. No evidence of teratogenicity with these drugs appeared in animal studies. Amprenavir and lopinavir have not yet been studied in pregnant women or neonates, although lopinavir is relatively well tolerated and provides potent ARV activity in heavily pretreated patients.[35]

MISCELLANEOUS AGENTS

Hydroxyurea used for myeloproliferative disorders and sickle cell anemia has potent teratogenic effects in animals. It should be avoided.[36]

CONCLUSION

Use of ARV prophylaxis with combination therapy is recommended for all pregnant women with HIV-1 infection regardless of antenatal HIV-1 RNA level. These women should be treated throughout pregnancy. They should be followed by a multidisciplinary team with careful, regular monitoring of the pregnancy and potential toxicities. No clinical evidence of adverse neurodevelopmental effects of ARV drugs is currently available.

REFERENCES

1. Taylor GP, Lyall EG, Mercey D, et al. British HIV Association guidelines for prescribing antiretroviral therapy in pregnancy (1998). *Sex Transm Infect* 1999;75:90–97.
2. Cooper ER, Charurat M, Mofenson L, et al. Combination antiretroviral strategies for the treatment of pregnant HIV-1-infected women and prevention of perinatal HIV-1 transmission. *J Acquir Immune Defic Syndr* 2002;29:484–494.
3. Public Health Service Task Force. Recommendations for use of antiretroviral drugs in pregnant HIV-1-infected women for maternal health and interventions to reduce perinatal HIV-1 transmission in the United States. Rockville, Md: AIDSinfo, US Department of Health and Human Services; 2003. Available at http://www.aidsinfo.nih.gov/guidelines. Accessed 2004 March 30.

4. Tuomala RE, Shapiro D, Mofenson LM, et al. Antiretroviral therapy during pregnancy and the risk of adverse outcome. *N Engl J Med* 2002;346: 1863–1870.

5. Connor EM, Sperling RS, Gelber R, et al. Reduction of maternal-infant transmission of human immunodeficiency virus type 1 with zidovudine treatment. Pediatric AIDS Clinical Trials Group Protocol 076 Study Group. *N Engl J Med* 1994;331:1173–1180.

6. Dybul M, Fauci AS, Bartlett JG, et al. Panel on Clinical Practices for the Treatment of HIV. Guidelines for using antiretroviral agents among HIV-infected adults and adolescents. Recommendations of the Panel on Clinical Practices for Treatment of HIV. *MMWR* 2002;51(RR-7):1–55.

7. Garcia-Tejedor A, Perales A, Maiques V. Protease inhibitor treatment in HIV pregnant women. Is it safe for newborns? *Int J Gynaecol Obstet* 2002; 76:175–176.

8. O'Sullivan MJ, Boyer PJ, Scott GB, et al. The pharmacokinetics and safety of zidovudine in the third trimester of pregnancy for women infected with human immunodeficiency virus and their infants: phase I acquired immunodeficiency syndrome clinical trials group study (protocol 082). Zidovudine Collaborative Working Group. *Am J Obstet Gynecol* 1993;168: 1510–1516.

9. Centers for Disease Control. Recommendations of the US Public Health Service Task Force on the use of zidovudine to reduce perinatal transmission of human immunodeficiency virus. *MMWR* 1994;43(RR-11):1–20.

10. Wade NA, Birkhead GS, Warren BL, et al. Abbreviated regimens of zidovudine prophylaxis and perinatal transmission of the human immunodeficiency virus. *N Engl J Med* 1998;339:1409–1414.

11. Shaffer N, Bulterys M, Simonds RJ. Short courses of zidovudine and perinatal transmission of HIV. *N Engl J Med* 1999;340:1042–1043.

12. Lambert JS, Watts DH, Mofenson L, et al. Risk factors for preterm birth, low birth weight, and intrauterine growth retardation in infants born to HIV-infected pregnant women receiving zidovudine. Pediatric AIDS Clinical Trials Group 185 Team. *AIDS* 2000;14:1389–1399.

13. Ioannidis JP, Abrams EJ, Ammann A, et al. Perinatal transmission of human immunodeficiency virus type 1 by pregnant women with RNA virus loads < 1000 copies/ml. *J Infect Dis* 2001;183:539–545.

14. Clarke SM, Mulcahy F, Healy CM, et al. The efficacy and tolerability of combination antiretroviral therapy in pregnancy: infant and maternal outcome. *Int J STD AIDS* 2000;11:220–223.

15. Orloff SL, Bulterys M, Vink P, et al. Maternal characteristics associated with antenatal, intrapartum, and neonatal zidovudine use in four US cities, 1994–1998. *J Acquir Immune Defic Syndr* 2001;28:65–72.

16. Mandelbrot L, Landreau-Mascaro A, Rekacewicz C, et al. Lamivudine-zidovudine combination for prevention of maternal-infant transmission of HIV-1. *JAMA* 2001;285:2083–2093.

17. Petra Study Team. Efficacy of three short-course regimens of zidovudine and lamivudine in preventing early and late transmission of HIV-1 from mother to child in Tanzania, South Africa, and Uganda (Petra study): a randomised, double-blind, placebo-controlled trial. *Lancet* 2002;359: 1178–1186.

18. Eshleman SH, Mracna M, Guay LA, et al. Selection and fading of resistance mutations in women and infants receiving nevirapine to prevent HIV-1 vertical transmission (HIVNET 012). *AIDS* 2001;15:1951–1957.

19. Koup RA, Brewster F, Grob P, et al. Nevirapine synergistically inhibits HIV-1 replication in combination with zidovudine, interferon or CD4 immunoadhesin. *AIDS* 1993;7:1181–1184.

20. Cunningham CK, Chaix ML, Rekacewicz C, et al. Development of resistance mutations in women receiving standard antiretroviral therapy who received intrapartum nevirapine to prevent perinatal human immunodeficiency virus type 1 transmission: a substudy of the pediatric AIDS clinical trials group protocol 316. *J Infect Dis* 2002;186:181–188.

21. Guay LA, Musoke P, Fleming T, et al. Intrapartum and neonatal single-dose nevirapine compared with zidovudine for prevention of mother-to-child transmission of HIV-1 in Kampala, Uganda: HIVNET 012 randomised trial. *Lancet* 1999;354:795–802.

22. Dorenbaum A, Cunningham CK, Gelber RD, et al. Two-dose intrapartum/newborn nevirapine and standard antiretroviral therapy to reduce perinatal HIV-1 transmission: a randomized trial. *JAMA* 2002;288: 189–198.

23. Gray J. HIV in the neonate. *J Hosp Infect* 1997;37:181–198.

24. Moodley J, Moodley D, Pillay K, et al. Pharmacokinetics and antiretroviral activity of lamivudine alone or when coadministered with zidovudine in human immunodeficiency virus type 1' infected pregnant women and their offspring. *J Infect Dis* 1998;178:1327–1333.

25. White A, Eldridge R, Andrews E. Birth outcomes following zidovudine exposure in pregnant women: the Antiretroviral Pregnancy Registry. *Acta Paediatr Suppl* 1997;421(Suppl. 1):86–88.

26. Culnane M, Fowler M, Lee SS, et al. Lack of long-term effects of in utero exposure to zidovudine among uninfected children born to HIV-1 infected women. Pediatric AIDS Clinical Trials Group Protocol 219/076 Teams. *JAMA* 1999;281:151–157.

27. Toltzis P, Mourton T, Magnuson T. Comparative embryonic cytotoxicity of European Collaborative Study. Exposure to antiretroviral therapy in utero or early life: the health of uninfected children born to HIV-infected women. *J Acquir Immune Defic Syndr* 2003;32:380–387.

28. Odinecs A, Nosbisch C, Keller RD, et al. In vivo maternal-fetal pharmacokinetics of stavudine (2?,3?-didehydro-3?-deoxythymidine) in pigtailed macaques (Macaca nemestrina). *Antimicrob Agents Chemother* 1996;40:196–202.

29. Easterbrook PJ, Waters A, Murad S, et al. Epidemiological risk factors for hypersensitivity reactions to abacavir. *HIV Med* 2003;4:321–324.

30. Arenas-Pinto A, Grant AD, Edwards S, et al. Lactic acidosis in HIV infected patients: a systematic review of published cases. *Sex Transm Infect* 2003;79:340–343.

31. Ibdah JA, Bennett MJ, Rinaldo P, et al. A fetal fatty-acid oxidation disorder as a cause of liver disease in pregnant women. *N Engl J Med* 1999; 340:1723–1731.

32. Ibdah JA, Yang Z, Bennett MJ. Liver disease in pregnancy and fetal fatty acid oxidation defects. *Mol Genet Metab* 2000;71:182–189.

33. Visnegarwala F, Krause KL, Musher DM. Severe diabetes associated with protease inhibitor therapy. *Ann Intern Med* 1997;127:947.
34. Eastone JA, Decker CF. New-onset diabetes mellitus associated with use of protease inhibitor. *Ann Intern Med* 1997;127:948.
35. Bulgheroni E, Citterio P, Croce F, et al. Analysis of protease inhibitor combinations in vitro: activity of lopinavir, amprenavir and tipranavir against HIV type wild-type and drug-resistance isolates. *J Antimicrob Chemother* 2004;53:464–468.
36. Aliverti V, Bonanomi L, Giavini E. Hydroxyurea as a reference standard in teratological screening. Comparison of the embryotoxic and teratogenic effects following single intraperitoneal or repeated oral administration to pregnant rats. *Arch Toxicol Suppl* 1980;4:239–247.

INDEX